MADNESS AND THE MILITARY

THE AUSTRALIAN ARMY HISTORY COLLECTION

Winning with Intelligence
Judy Thomas

Duntroon
Darren Moore

The Warrior Poets
Robert Morrison

The History of the Royal Australian Corps of Transport 1973–2000
Albert Palazzo

Defenders of Australia
Albert Palazzo

The Fight Leaders
D. Butler, A. Argent and J. Shelton

Operation Orders
Pat Beale

Little by Little
Michael Tyquin

Red Coats to Cams: A History of Australian Infantry 1788 to 2001
Ian Kuring

Bowler of Gallipoli: Witness to the Anzac Legend
Frank Glen

Vets at War
Ian M. Parsonson

Only One River to Cross: An Australian Soldier Behind Enemy Lines in Korea
A.M. Harris

The Fragile Forts: The Fixed Defences of Sydney Harbour 1788-1963
Peter Oppenheim

Hassett—Australian Leader
John Essex-Clark

Never Late—The 2/9th Australian Infantry Battalion
Gordon Dickens

This collection is a joint-venture between the
Australian Army History Unit and
Australian Military History Publications

MADNESS AND THE MILITARY

AUSTRALIA'S EXPERIENCE OF THE GREAT WAR

MICHAEL TYQUIN

2006

First published in Australia – 2006
by AUSTRALIAN MILITARY HISTORY PUBLICATIONS.
13 Veronica Place, Loftus 2232 Australia.
Phone: 02-9542-6771 Fax: 02-9542-6787
Website: www.warbooks.com.au

Written by: Michael Tyquin

Printed in Australia by Shannon Books Pty Ltd – Victoria.
Typesetting: Margaret McNally, Canberra
and Typesmith Pty Ltd, Carlton NSW.
Cover Design: Michael Tyquin.

National Library of Australia – ISBN: 1876 439 890

DEDICATION

Dedicated to the 'no-hopers', the loners, the disenfranchised servicemen and women and their families who suffered in silence as a result of the Great War.

I knew a simple soldier boy
Who grinned at life in empty joy,
Slept soundly through the lonesome dark,
And whistled early with the lark.

In winter trenches, cowed and glum,
With crumps and lice and lack of rum,
He put a bullet through his brain,
No one spoke of him again.

You smug-faced crowds with kindling eye
Who cheer when soldier lads march by,
Sneak home and pray you'll never know
The hell where youth and laughter go.

Siegfried Sassoon

CONTENTS

List of Photographs

Preface

In many respects *Madness and the Military* is a logical sequel to my previous work which dealt with the Australian Army medical services and an earlier assessment of the medical problems of Gallipoli in 1915. 'Madness' is not used pejoratively here; rather I have employed it to give a sense of the 'madness' of war in the context of neurosis and to give 'shell shock' an added dimension to the uncertainty surrounding its diagnosis and treatment in 1914–1918.[1] In reading numerous soldiers' diaries and letters it was obvious that, in at least some of their writing, both at Gallipoli and later in France, they were expressing severe emotional and psychological problems. The Western Front and its associated horrors still have a firm hold on the popular imagination. The period 1914–1918 in France and Belgium is a byword for wanton slaughter and terror of nightmarish proportions and many books have been written about all aspects of that war. However the bulk of such scholarship continues to focus on strategy and individual commanders. This is unfortunate as it has ignored a core part of the individual experience of war—to fight in it and to suffer from it in a very personal way. To the extent that the focus on strategy and tactics has ignored common experiences, it has denied us a better understanding of shell shock.[2] As George Mosse has shown, for the cultural historian 'shell shock provides an excellent example of the fusion of medical diagnosis and social prejudice, which had taken place during the previous century and a half. Shell-shock, in reality, was not as vague a disease as it seemed at the time; rather, as we look upon the phenomenon from a historical perspective, it was an injury, which, while raising disturbing medical questions, was easily co-opted by traditional cultural prejudice which, so it was thought, could provide it with a readily understood context.'[3] The whole episode of war neurosis from this time is one of the few uncharted areas of Australia's military history.

We still seek answers to what happened in the Great War and why it commands such a pivotal place in Western memory. Apart from the various officially sanctioned and vetted official histories—medical and otherwise—its psychological casualties have been largely ignored. More importantly for

Australian society and military and cultural historiography, the mental casualties of that conflagration have been largely forgotten. While every city and town has its shrine of commemoration, nowhere on their gilded or marbled exteriors are the 'shell shocked' recorded or acknowledged for what they were—the mental debris of the war. While there may be cracks in these stone edifices, no human failures are admitted to these holy sanctuaries.

To some extent this 'omission' has been deliberately orchestrated. At the end of the war society wanted to forget and to move on. To assist in this process and to find a suitable image for the new nation (Australia became federated only twelve years before the outbreak of war), the gifted journalist C.E.W. Bean—who recorded much of Australia's contribution to the war—manufactured an Australian icon: the Anzac 'digger'. While there is now a view held by some that Australian commemoration of war as 'tradition' encompasses both a private (digger) and a public (Anzac) dimension, the substance of *Madness and the Military* overarches both.[4]

Laconic, tough, resourceful, but above all masculine, this idealised image endures today as part of the (male) Australian perception of itself. Those soldiers who succumbed to mental illness were not part of Bean's New World. They had failed to make the grade and, while initially they were included in the nation's pantheon of heroes, they were the first to fall victim to cynicism and budgetary constraints before being quietly forgotten as the country moved towards the 1930s and on to another social cataclysm. True, returned services organisations lobbied on behalf of their psychologically scarred colleagues, as happened in Britain and New Zealand, but mainstream society increasingly found these men a burden. Then, as the country teetered towards economic ruin in the 'Great Depression', even closer scrutiny was placed on the legitimacy of their suffering and on their pension entitlements. Once again, comparisons which had been made early in the war were drawn between the shell shocked and the malingerer.

These men who had failed morally and mentally could not hope to meet the expectations of the jingoistic Australia of the interwar years, let alone face their families and friends as returned warriors. They had been unmanned through succumbing to fear or the other horrors of war. The great tragedy for these soldiers was that they experienced this type of trauma at a time when modern warfare had the technology to produce unprecedented killing power, but while the science of psychology was still in its infancy. Men with war neuroses would have to struggle against the scepticism of the military, confusion in medical circles, and the perceived link between mental illness and moral weakness—even degeneracy, made by the wider society.

Readers are entitled to question the presence of so much contemporary British material in what purports to be an Australian study of shell shock. For the period under review, both the Australian military and the civilian and army medical establishments were not only based and formed along imperial lines, but continued to use British Army doctrine and medical and scientific mores and developments as did other British dominions. Members of both armies were subjected to the same war, the same conditions and horrors, largely shared a common Anglo-Saxon cultural inheritance and were usually treated (at least until 1919) in the same 'specialist' institutions at the front and in Great Britain. It is really not until the early twenties that differences appear in the way the two nations viewed and treated their psychological war casualties. There is much material and further theses to be found and researched in this area of military history, particularly for the interwar period in Australia, which so often has been dismissed as an historical backwater. I hope this work will encourage others to take up that challenge.

Those looking for the sometimes lurid photographs in works that purport to tell the psychological side of conflict will be disappointed. The lack of clinical photos reflects the delicacy about mental illness that prevailed even in wartime. While many images of casualties, their wounds and subsequent surgery, were reproduced in both the Australian official and medical histories of the war, nothing has survived, assuming photographs were taken, of psychological casualties. This is in contrast to the British experience in which even the *Times Illustrated History* of the war reproduced photographs (innocuous enough) for its coverage of shell shock for its readers.

I would like to record my special thanks to colleagues and medical historians Dr Bryan Egan in Melbourne and Dr Peter Barham—author of *Forgotten Lunatics of the Great War*—in the United Kingdom, for their valuable comments on the first drafts of this work. Miss Brenda Heagney, as always, was a cheerful and obliging font of wisdom and directed me to a number of sources. I would also like to acknowledge Mr Neil Sharkey and Mr Simeon Barlow of the Canberra and Sydney offices of the National Archives of Australia; and Mr. David Joliffe and the research centre staff of the Australian War Memorial, Canberra, for their assistance with archival material and records. Miss Alyson Dalby, librarian of the Royal Australasian College of Physicians, was gracious in offering me the facilities of that library. I acknowledge the generous permission of Dr Richard Lindstrom to quote from his doctoral thesis on the subject of psychological casualties. The staff at the Kingston repository of the State Records of New South Wales were also most helpful with documents relating to Broughton Hall Asylum and its former patients, as was the New South Wales Health Department in granting access to its case notes. I record my special thanks for the encouragement given me by Mr Roger Lee, Head of the Army History Unit in Canberra and to colleague Professor John Pearn and Emma Robertson. The manuscript was enhanced as a result of Cathy McCullagh's editing skills. As always, Mr Clive Baker proved an unflappable collaborator in the publication of this book. The completion of this work was assisted by a grant from the Department of Veterans' Affairs.[5]

Endnotes

1 Robert Kosky has written of the place of asylums within society's views of madness: 'The intellectual relocation of madness within society as a whole, without the separating constraints imposed by the asylum, may have great repercussions in popular perceptions of madness. We have come to accept as truth that the stigmatisation of the mad and the fear of mental illness generally found in the community is a *sine qua non* associated with insanity, that they are inherent responses of rational humans to the irrational.' From 'Morality to Madness: A Reappraisal of the Asylum Movement in Psychiatry 1800–1940', *Australian and New Zealand Journal of Psychiatry*, vol. 20, 1986, p.187.

2 Curiously though, it has also been asserted that 'shell shock now stands at the centre of the Great War narrative.' Fiona Reid, 'Playing the Game to the Army: The Royal Army Medical Corps, Shell Shock and the Great War', in *War & Society*, vol. 23, no.1, May 2005, p. 61. This is a strange piece of post-modernist scholarship in which there is no reference to, or critique of, the British official medical history.

3 George Mosse, 'Shell-shock as Social Disease', *Journal of Contemporary History*, 35 (1), 2000, p.101.

4 Graham Seal, *Inventing Anzac: The Digger and National Mythology*, University of Queensland, 2004, pp. 3–4.

5 The author wishes to acknowledge the support of the Australian Government Department of Veterans' Affairs which provided a grant to assist publication under the Australian Government's commemorations program *Saluting their Service*. The following disclaimer applies: The Department of Veterans' Affairs has not participated in the research or production or exercised editorial control over the work's contents, and the views expressed and the conclusions reached herein do not necessarily represent those of the Commonwealth which expressly disclaims any responsibility for the content or accuracy of the work.

Acronyms and Abbreviations

'Repat'	(Australian) repatriation system
AAH	Australian Auxiliary Hospital
AAMC	Australian Army Medical Corps
AGH	Australian General Hospital
AIF	Australian Imperial Force
ANZAC (Anzac)	Australian and New Zealand Army Corps
BEF	British Expeditionary Force
CCS	Casualty Clearing Station
DAH	Disordered Action of the Heart
DDMS	Deputy Director of Medical Services
DGMS	Director General Medical Services
DOW	Died of Wounds
ES & SILA	Ex-Sailors and Soldiers Imperial League of Australia
GPI	General Paralysis of Insane
KIA	Killed in Action
NYDN (W)	Shell shock with wound
NYDN	Not Yet Diagnosed (Nervous?)
NYDN (S)	Shell shock no wound
PTSD/S	Post Traumatic Stress Disorder/Syndrome
RAMC	Royal Army Medical Corps
RMO	Regimental Medical Officer

Glossary of Terminology

RSA – Returned Soldiers Association which changed its name in 1940 to the Returned Soldiers, Sailors & Airmen's Imperial League of Australia, which in turn evolved into the Returned Services League in 1965 and which, from 1990, became known as the Returned and Services League.

Abreaction – the dissipation of emotion by reviving it and reliving the experience which originally evoked it; the free expression and release of repressed emotion.

Alienists – psychologists.

Anzac Day – Australian national celebration dating from the 1930s held on 25 April each year in commemoration of the landings on the beaches of the Gallipoli Peninsula in 1915.

Aphonia – inability to speak above a whisper.

Association of Ideas – ideas tend to evoke other ideas that are related by similarity, contrast, contiguity in space or time, etc.

Commotional shock – concussion due to direct physical injury.

Conversion Hysteria – those hysterical states in which the mechanism of conversion dominates.

'Digger' – a popular term for the Australian soldier, applied especially to infantrymen.

Effort Syndrome – nervous and heart disturbances associated with normal fear reaction.

Faradism – the use of interrupted or faradic current (electricity).

Functional – contrasted with organic; functional disorders are those in which there is no structural damage; compare hysterical paralysis with organic paralysis following apoplexy.

Hysteria – a nervous disorder in which the solution of emotional conflict is formed by the unconscious simulation of disease.

Mutism – inability or refusal to speak.

Neurasthenia – a nervous disorder characterised by ideas of weakness and morbid feelings of fatigue.

Neurosis – a nervous disorder; when anxiety predominates this is termed 'anxiety neurosis'; when obsessions are a feature, it is referred to as 'obsessional neurosis.'

Persuasion – a method of treatment in which the patient is induced to accept an idea after reasoning.

Psychoanalysis – any manoeuvre for bringing buried thoughts into consciousness.

Psychoneurosis – a nervous disorder intermediate in gravity between neurosis and psychosis.

Psychosis – a major disorder of the mind; the important psychoses are: schizophrenia, manic-depressive psychosis, and paraphrenia.

PTSD/S – Post Traumatic Stress Disorder/Syndrome.

Somatic – relating to the body rather than to the mind.

Suggestion - the implantation of an idea without exercise of critical judgement.

Chapter One

Introduction

Shell shock is one of the enduring metaphors for the experience of the Western Front between 1914 and 1918. It 'was one of the most widespread battlefield injuries during the First World War: it seemed unlike any of the other wounds contracted in the war, an injury without any bodily signs, a mass outbreak of mental disorder.'[1] From the Australian perspective, it is not widely known that shell-shocked soldiers were a feature of the Gallipoli campaign, a full year before the men of the First Australian Imperial Force (AIF) participated in the European theatre of the war. Similarly, a percentage of soldiers who were treated for various mental illnesses either never left Australia or never fired a shot when they did go overseas. To a degree then, that other great image of World War I—'no man's land'—is almost an allegory for servicemen's mental health in Australia and the attitudes of the government, the military and medicine in the first decades of the twentieth century.

While most unit histories of the AIF contain casualty figures, stories of daring-do, battle plans and the trials and tribulations of their members, they are almost totally silent on the matter of psychological stress or mental breakdown within their own ranks. A surprising number of surviving private diaries also pass over killing, self-doubt or cowardice, although there is a significant portion that does relate the writer's personal terror or inability to really come to terms with his wartime experiences. Shell shock was not only unnerving—it was 'new'. It differed from other diseases and 'it emerged during a singular period of social change, accelerated by the First World War, when relationships between individual citizens and bureaucratic institutions were in flux (especially those between the army, soldiers, military doctors, mental hospitals, and those on the home front).'[2]

Despite the vastly better understanding of psychological aspects of mankind nowadays, any attempt to analyse war neuroses from a perspective eighty years removed is daunting. 'The meanings that we ascribe to shell shock today are difficult to disentangle from the events that took place during the war, and from the amalgam of meanings [of shell shock] that have grown through the years.'[3] Modern-day readers will also be conscious of Post Traumatic Stress Disorder/

Syndrome (PTSD/S), which some have seen as the successor of the shell shock of earlier times. Reference will be made to PTSD later in this book. The unenviable position of the average regimental medical officer (RMO) at the front, who was not only recently a civilian but also generally untutored in the ways of mental health, is readily appreciated

Death, of course, is a common theme in most soldiers' personal accounts. But thoughts of killing, the readiness or otherwise to do it, and the consequences of killing, remain as suppressed as they were in the minds of the men (and a few women, usually nurses) who wrote these often pathetic glimpses into hell. The much-lauded work of journalist Charles Bean, author of Australia's official history of World War I and arguably the creator of the Anzac[4] 'myth', also shied away from the issue of mental illness in the war. Even Colonel Arthur Graham Butler, DSO, himself an otherwise compassionate front-line medical officer, could still write an official medical history in which he all but condemned the neuroses of ex-servicemen as either symptomatic of weakness or as borderline malingering.

Subsequent generations of unquestioning Australians have largely been content with this view ever since. Scholars have variously cited Alistair Thompson and his argument that 'as the public myth of the [Gallipoli] campaign was used to promote the idea of Australia's birth, it became remote to some participants, who in turn recomposed their recollections of the war to match popular memory.'[5] More recently, others have proposed that the digger culture is a 'private' tradition developed by 'a highly *specialised* group of *primarily youthful males* [emphasis added].'[6] This sort of claim is unsubstantiated and is couched in the cant of 'our boys' still used today when politicians and others either laud soldiers when successful or commiserate with casualties and grieving relatives when they are not. Descriptions such as this continue to deny the existence of war neuroses—of those outside that charmed fraternity of invulnerable youth.

These mentally scarred men could not therefore enjoy a sanctioned place in the young nation's idealised archetype of bronzed, hypo-masculine warrior. The icon could accommodate the physically wounded, the larrikin and the ill-disciplined; but it denied a place to the mentally scarred in the new nation's pantheon. Those who suffered from war neuroses were also left out and, in many cases, these men were doomed to suffer silently for decades. The 'shell shocked' whose various eccentricities were whispered about in lounge rooms and pubs around the country, could not hope to match the expectations required of the war hero whose attributes were being manufactured even while they were repatriated to Australia. To the extent that they could not even begin to meet these expectations, their downward spiral into despair only accelerated.

Media commentators of the twenty-first century still perfuse Anzac and Remembrance Day ceremonies in Australia with a litany of insipid reminiscences, drawing on half memories of what was never a real reflection of the men and women who served in that first AIF. There are no blemishes, there is no whisper of mental or emotional breakdown. The Anzacs or 'diggers' (as these soldiers came to be known) are in every sense the nation's finest. Certainly there could be no recognition of the thousands of mentally broken warriors who returned home in 1918 and 1919. They suffered in silence or saw their marriages or families broken up in a ghastly melange of recurrent nightmares, domestic violence, alcoholism, or suicide. There are probably thousands of personal tragedies that will never be known to us. As one commentator has demonstrated 'psychological disorder was one of the war's least obvious but most devastating consequences.'[7]

Even recent historical research in Australia provides scant recognition of mental illnesses seen during 1914–1918.[8] Joy Damousi's *Freud in the Antipodes: A Cultural History of Psychology in Australia* (2005) is the only work that attempts to look at shell shock, albeit it as part of a broader cultural canvas.[9] More recently, some refreshing work has emerged in Britain which looks at this less glamorous side of the Great War. Peter Barham's insightful *Forgotten Lunatics of the Great War* (2004) is a good example of a detailed foray into this field as is George Mosse's article on shell shock in the *Journal of Contemporary History* (2000). Otherwise, the focus in so far as it falls on psychological casualties has been on more recent conflicts: World War II, Vietnam and the Gulf Wars, with their accompanying terminologies such as 'combat stress' and 'PTSD'. In this vein John Raftery's *Marks of War* (2003) finally addresses aspects of the war neuroses from Australia's Pacific War, while Brendan O'Keefe in *Medicine at War: Medical Aspects of Australia's Involvement in Southeast Asian Conflicts 1950–1972* (1994) looked at other stressors.

Other published scholarship, at least in Australia, does not mention shell shock or neuroses, including those works that specifically deal with the war or postwar periods. This corpus of work includes Richard Waterhouse's *Vision Splendid: A Social and Cultural History of Rural Australia* (2005), John McQuilton's *Rural Australia and the Great War* (2001) and Robert Kearney's *Silent Voices: The Story of the 12th Battalion in Australia, Egypt, Gallipoli, France and Belgium during the Great War 1914–1918* (2005) to name but a few. Even books in which the theme of the war-damaged soldier might be thought to be central, ignore the issue. For example, *The Last Shilling: A History of Repatriation in Australia* (1994) by C. Lloyd and J. Rees barely mentions mental illness or the neurotic ex-soldier. Similarly Joy Damousi's earlier work *The Labour of Loss:*

Mourning, Memory and Wartime (1999) and C. Coleburne and D. Makinnon's work *Madness in Australia: Histories, Heritage and Asylum* (2003) offer only fleeting references. Michael McKernan's *The Australian People and the Great War* (1980), while sympathetic, only offers a few glimpses into disillusioned dreams and shattered family lives. Dale Blair's *Dinkum Diggers: an Australian Battalion* (2001) touches upon suicide and the breakdown of 'digger durability'. A. G. Owen in M. Nixon and R. Taft (eds.), *Psychology in Australia: Achievements and Prospects* (1977) wrote specifically of psychology and the Australian armed forces but did not allude to shell shock or World War I at all.

Bill Gammage's seminal work *The Broken Years* (1974) refers to the problem but does not pursue it despite its centrality to the title of his book. There are, however, glimpses into the dark underside of the waggish Aussie soldier. We can also see hints in *The Limits of Hope*, Marilyn Lake's work on soldier settlement in Victoria between the wars.[10] In Australian literature, *My Brother Jack* (1967) by George Johnston and Graham McInnes's *Road to Gundagai* (1970) are the best examples, but there has been nothing of the genre made famous by British author Pat Barker in her *Regeneration* trilogy. Writing in 1985 Jane Ross observed that 'the fighting digger of Anzac remains an integral part of our national experience' and she called for a more balanced approach to the history of the digger before proceeding to look at the main components of the Anzac myth.[11] However the potential for war neurosis to challenge that myth has not been addressed.

Some readers will relate to the reticence of older relatives to talk about their wartime experiences. This was particularly so for the generation that fought in the Great War. This reluctance may have been 'a way of protecting a traumatised self but it was not just an individual act. It was part of a larger national act of submerging experiences of violence. This history has generally been closed to wives and children, who were not allowed into the inner world of veterans at any time, even in the reminiscences of later years.'[12] I would argue otherwise, that wives and children of war neurotics *were* intimately associated with this history. *Madness and the Military* attempts to shed some light on this closed world of shadows and nightmares, if only to explain why and how psychologically afflicted soldiers coped, or did not cope, on their return home.

What follows is not meant to be a clinical psychological study of neurotic soldiers and veterans from World War I. Historians are now 'aware that the problem of [mental] trauma does not lend itself to any dogmatic interpretation.'[13] Rather, the aim is to record some part of the forgotten history of a generation of soldiers who, because medicine and the military viewed them as somehow morally inferior or genetically prone to neurosis, have been effectively locked out of our collective memory of war as it is now celebrated. It is also a plea to Australia to honour its war dead, not as the bronzed Anzac, but by way of an infinitely more complex icon, in men and women who were good and bad, heroic and fragile, and to include the weak and unlucky amongst them. The book is unashamedly gender specific, as few females (who were mainly nurses; and indeed some of these women were deeply traumatised) were as directly affected, or exposed to the horrors, real or imagined, of wartime service. This said, it will be shown that numbers of male soldiers who never saw a shot fired suffered neuroses, as did others who never left the shores of Australia.

An attempt is made to recreate some aspects of front-line fighting so as to provide the reader with a point of reference against which to measure subsequent chapters. This includes the mechanisms of injury, both physical and psychological, and the official military and medical views of war neuroses, particularly the origins of a phrase that entered the English language for the first time: 'shell shock'. Chapter three sets the scene by analysing the difficulty posed to both the military and medicine in appreciating shell shock as a legitimate human condition, followed by a discussion of the suspicion of malingering that always seems to have accompanied afflicted soldiers. Chapter four looks at the World War and the individual soldier's place in that conflict.[14] The image of the shell-shocked soldier is at once both supremely individual and yet representative of an entire generation. In chapter five we look at contemporary methods for treating soldiers diagnosed with shell shock. The subsequent chapter analyses the response of the military which struggled to deal with what many senior officers saw as malingering, while insisting that discipline and the war effort had to be maintained at all costs.

Chapter seven provides some insights into the reaction of Australian society and its attitude to the shell-shocked soldier. This includes important groups in the overall management, clinical or otherwise, of these soldiers such as the Defence and Repatriation departments, soldiers' families, the press, returned service organisations and the courts. We offer some insights into mainstream medicine in Australia and abroad during and after the war, and the progress of psychology in spite of the uncertainty of the science, together with the different schools of thought that flourished throughout and following the war. There follows a description of the evolution of types of treatment and management in the field and, importantly, the various state lunatic authorities. Chapter eight focuses specifically on the postwar, and what might be regarded as a 'lost' generation. We will look briefly at the evolution of psychology in Australia, particularly in the 1920s. A number of case studies of soldiers, presented to illustrate how they coped with their demons, will be revisited. This is an attempt to provide an overarching synthesis between point of injury and subsequent treatment of soldiers, together with the consequences for these individuals.

The final chapter is a series of observations that concludes with the thesis that the 'no man's land' of popular memory might serve as a metaphor for the state of men's minds between 1914 and 1918. To a lesser degree, the wilderness and danger implied by the imagery of no man's land might as well describe the uncertainties of military psychiatry at the time.

Endnotes

1 Mosse, 'Shell-shock as Social Disease', p.101.

2 C. Feudtner, 'Minds the Dead Have Ravished: Shell Shock, History and the Evolution of Disease Systems', *History of Science*, 31, Part 4, no.94, 1993, p. 379.

3 Peter Leese, *Shell Shock: Traumatic Neurosis and the British Soldiers of the First World War*, London, 2002, p. 161.

4 ANZAC is the acronym used for those men who served in the Australian and New Zealand Army Corps. Common usage has seen the acronym now accepted as 'Anzac'.

5 Leese, *Shell Shock*, p. 173.

6 Seal, *Inventing Anzac*, p. 63. At enlistment, those aged between 18 and 21 made up only 11.37 per cent of the AIF, while those at the other end of the scale, i.e. men aged between 37 and 45, constituted 12.28 per cent. A.G. Butler, *Official History of the Australian Army Medical Services in the War of 1914–1918, Special Problems and Services*, vol. III, Australian War Memorial, Canberra, 1943, pp. 898–9.

7 Richard Lindstrom, 'The Australian Experience of Psychological Casualties in War 1915–1939', thesis submitted for the Degree of Doctor of Philosophy, Department of Humanities, Faculty of Arts, Victoria University of Technology, February 1997, p. 5.

8 The only exception is Richard Lindstrom's outstandingly detailed and insightful, but unfortunately still unpublished, 1997 doctoral thesis on the subject.

9 In an earlier work, *Living with the Aftermath*, (2001), Damousi presented a comprehensive analysis of the Second World War, with a few references to World War I.

10 Marilyn Lake, *The Limits of Hope: Soldier Settlement in Victoria 1915–1938*, Oxford University Press, Melbourne, 1987.

11 Jane Ross, *The Myth of the Digger: The Australian Soldier in Two World Wars*, Hale & Iremonger, Sydney, 1985, p. 12.

12 John Raftery, *Marks of War*, Lythrum Press, Adelaide, 2003, p. xvii.

13 Simon Wessely reviewing Paul Lerner's 'Hysterical Men: War, Psychiatry and the Politics of Germany 1890–1930', *History of Psychiatry*, vol.15, Issue 4, no.60, December 2004, p. 490.

14 The usual convention of disguising real names, especially of patients, has been followed, except where names have previously been identified in the public domain, through published articles, the newspapers, etc.

Chapter Two

Background

Much has been made of World War I as the first major conflict of the industrial age. The place of technology is now regarded as a key factor in events leading to 1914 as 'the accumulated explosive power that advanced science had developed was concentrated on the goal of mass destruction.'[1] By this time the world had already witnessed such conflicts as the civil war in the United States, the Franco–Prussian War and the Russo–Japanese War of 1905.[2] All these conflicts had, to a larger or lesser extent, involved mass production, and their strategists and commanders had been influenced in their calculations by the first rumblings of industrialisation as it affected transport and munitions.

Since 1918 writers have focused on the impersonal, machine-driven nature of that war in their search for the origins of 'shell shock', a phrase first used by army doctors in 1914 to make sense of otherwise inexplicable mental disability and breakdown on the battlefield. It was not long before this industrialised aspect of modern warfare was being posited as *the* major cause of the condition. As some scholars have argued, 'Neurosis was a psychic effect not of war but of industrialised war in particular.'[3] Others have suggested that our 'natural' desire to elevate the individual above the meaningless and impersonal aspect of mechanised war is actually a response to this depersonalisation of conflict. This appears to be borne out in the primacy of Anzac Day in the Australian calendar. Anzac Day is accorded a particular reverence which reflects the attempts of people to understand a massive war in which the age-old myths of the warrior are still accorded a place in that juggernaut of deadly armaments and cold hard steel.

The place of shell shock in the First World War and its very novelty have been eloquently summarised by author Stephen Garton who suggests that 'the intensity of modern warfare (the large numbers of combatants), the vastly destructive capacity of weapons (particularly shells, grenades, and later, automatic weapons), the protracted nature of the conflict...and the relative passivity of modern warfare (with soldiers being subjected to long periods of shelling and gunfire from unseen forces) created unique conditions for an increased incidence of stress and psychological breakdown.'[4] This attempt at making 'sense' of a situation so utterly beyond their control would have been profoundly more difficult for young men in 1914 who had been raised on romantic and nationalistic stories of war which were invariably short, often honourable, but always sanitised in the telling to avoid the less glamorous side of war. Historians and others, in analysing the collective memory of that war, still concentrate on the physical. 'The manly adventure which had disfigured the men was, during the 1920s, lauded as heroic and glorious by the likes of C.E.W. Bean and others.' The soldiers' twisted bodies became synonymous with sacrifice, deserving of the adulation that would be compensation for their loss. Their 'desire for affirmation and self-esteem coalesced around celebrations on Anzac Day with a recognition of that [physical] disability.'[5] But there is no mention here of contorted or convulsed minds or psyche.

We should note the relative infancy of the science of psychology and psychiatry in the period under review. The situation at the end of 1918 was summarised by an official historian at the time: 'Shell-shock was a term used in the early days to describe a variety of conditions ranging from cowardice to maniacal insanity. After endless discussion the physicians and metaphysicians, the psychologists, physiologists, and neurologists *invented* [emphasis added] a series of names which did not leave the matter much clearer than it was when they found it.'[6] In 1917 an American medical officer in Britain reported to his superiors the prediction that 'the wide prevalence of neuroses among soldiers will direct attention to the fact that this kind of illness has been almost wholly ignored while great advances have been made in the treatment of all others.'[7] As in British psychiatry, the few medical practitioners in Australia who at the turn of the century had 'specialised' in mental illness 'found that their genuine desire to ensure people who suffered from elusive neurotic ailments was nullified in large part by the doctors' own endeavours.' They wanted their patients 'to be at once autonomous and connected by meaningful ties to the social community, but their intrusive morality defined both the autonomy and the social bonds in that narrow, restrictive manner. Freedom, in their vocabulary, tended to mean little more than self-control, while their vision of healthy social intercourse revealed the prejudices of their class and gender.'[8] This 'intrusive morality' was shared by those who would not only lead troops in battle, but by those who treated their symptoms, and later, by others who would deprive them of their place in the history of the Great War. Morality, specifically that of the Edwardian middle class in both England and Australia, is a thread that runs through the discussion of shell shock. The whole endeavour to manage these men was bedevilled by the relatively primitive state of medicine and psychology at the time and indeed it was not until the1980s that 'the psychological sequelae of traumatisation in war were more fully appreciated.'[9]

In 1915 it was not possible to correctly diagnose and treat the thousands of men who suffered from war neuroses that are often grouped under the ubiquitous catch-all of 'shell shock'. A key point of disagreement was how these nervous breakdowns came about: 'Were they a product of the excessive stress of war, a stress sufficient to weaken even the soundest psychological constitution, or were there some inherent faults in these men that meant that some succumbed to shell-shock while others survived mentally unscathed?'[10] Medicine and the military struggled for answers well into the 1930s. The other theme to be examined here is the military's suspicion, never far below the surface, that war neuroses were a deliberate individual threat to authority, discipline and even the war effort itself. It was left to medicine to ponder on the implied threat to national pride in the unmanning of its soldiers. Given the British Edwardian (and German Wilhelmine) social and cultural mores of those times, contemporary writing inevitably linked soldiers' mental states with morality. By association this also suggested a link with malingering and that scourge of army discipline—self-inflicted wounds.

But the mental trauma of war experiences did not necessarily give way to a comfortable return to 'normality'. One of the themes to be addressed in this book is the response of Australian society to the issues and, specifically, to those soldiers afflicted with neuroses. There is almost a cultural divide within the country between a genuine sympathy that did not fit with the military's view and, later, an artificial construct of the new nation's identity which offered no refuge to its mentally 'weak'. Within the longed-for safety of Australia's quiet and predictable domesticity, the war neurotic fell from grace as the cheers of welcome died away. By the twenties some veterans would become pariahs; others were seen as a burden on the state; while some ex-soldiers became an embarrassment, if not a real physical threat to either themselves or their families. Perhaps those incurables who found a home in asylums had the best of it. This situation reflected the British experience in which the body eventually became the conduit for psychological stress. 'How men outside the official treatment network survived has largely gone unrecorded, though one suggestion is that their distressed mental state converted into physical symptoms such as debility, anaemia, gastritis or rheumatism.'[11] Generally these men had given up any hope of participation in the postwar nation—one fit only for heroes of the new Anzac myth. Despite the much-vaunted larrikinism and casualness of the Australian psyche, in reality there was little room for personal failure in war.

The importance of language, in particular the English language, not only in the genesis of 'shell shock' but as an explanation for its longevity, should not be underestimated. Like the foul, greasy trench mud of Flanders, the phrase has stuck and it remains even today a potent symbol of the human dimension of war.[12] 'Through the language of mental conflicts and dark unconscious forces...the inner drama could enter the public realm and draw on the fear, guilt, and pathos of the European conflict. Shell shock came to symbolize the valour and romance of battles lost.'[13] The official Australian medical historian of World War I, Arthur Butler, offered his own suggestion of its origin: 'Whether the term or the concept "shell shock" came first from the medical service or from the soldiers themselves will probably never be known—possibly medical officers adopted almost unconsciously a soldier's phrase which fitted the novel phenomena.'[14] Whatever the case, the phrase was civilianised and subsequently passed into the vernacular to describe people who were 'stunned' or 'shattered' on the battlefield. There lies within the term, though, an implied weakness or vulnerability—one that did not sit well with an Australian military intent to show that it was as good as the armies of the Old World.

It has been noted elsewhere that the phrase also described 'a kind of English genius of linguistic compression, in which a host of allusions are fused into two simple vertical syllables'. Neither the Germans nor the French had anything like it—'the German *Kreigshysterie Granatshock*, and the French *choc traumatique* don't quite have the same phonetic ring even though they reflect meaning just as precisely.'[15] As the guns of the Second World War heralded the return to conflict, another explanation, current as early as 1914, was revisited to explain the success of 'shell shock' as a stock phrase in the English-speaking world. It was 'supposed that that these patients had all received injuries to their central nervous systems, small haemorrhages, small lacerations, and the name shell-shock was coined. Being of good alliterative quality it caught on.'[16]

While doubtful of its etymology, Butler was unambiguous in his own view of the phenomenon. 'The term had been in use for some time and was *loosely* applied to all cases of physical and mental breakdown within the battle zone without apparent wound. It had become indeed a *diagnostic shibboleth and an open sesame* [emphasis added] to the Base [i.e. a safe area].'[17] As we shall see, this is a view that coloured his subsequent treatment of war neuroses in his published history and was also one never far from the views of the Australian military. Those, like Butler, who took a moral view of war neurosis 'were inclined to read the symptom back into a biological or familial degeneracy. The neurotic symptom, which the war merely made overt, was rooted in inherited abnormalities.'[18] Unfortunately for the victims, the tendency to drape psychological diagnoses with morality (sometimes identified by social class) did a disservice to the very people military medicine was trying to help.

Throughout Butler's accounts of World War I there is an element of doubt and more than a hint of disdain for the 'weak' male who failed the ultimate test of war. Like many of his contemporaries, the journalist C.E.W. Bean and senior Australian commanders included, Butler's public school background, unshakeable middle-class morality and Anglo-Saxon cultural heritage meant that he was scarcely able to conceal the unease, if not contempt, for the stigma that attached to the military psychological casualty. In this he was a man of his times and cannot be judged too harshly. In Edwardian society there was something almost effeminate in the hysterical male. Indeed hitherto this condition had been considered in medical circles as an exclusively female manifestation.[19] 'The efficacy of the term "shell-shock" lay in its power to provide a masculine sounding substitute for the effeminate associations of "hysteria" and to disguise the troubling parallels between male war neurosis and the female nervous disorders epidemic [sic] before the war.'[20] This then was a fundamental jolt to wartime society. The consequences were obvious. 'If the essence of manliness was not to complain, then shell-shock was the body language of masculine complaint, a disguised male protest not only against the war but against the concept of "manliness" itself.'[21] Any femininity in the Australian soldier had to be excised not only by officialdom but by the men themselves if any sort of acceptable public image was to be espoused either during the war or after it. Private writings, diaries, poems and even 'official' paintings and sketches testify to feelings of tenderness, compassion or grief among Australian soldiers to their comrades. But Charles Bean, too, had airbrushed these traits, even from the old bush myth on which he was basing his idealised society. This left a hard, but acceptable, core of 'male' attributes.

There was a contradiction here that worked to the shell-shocked soldier's advantage—at least in the short term. With the popular acceptance early in the war of the term 'shell shock', 'victims of neurosis were accorded the regard and sympathy that should be reserved for the physically disabled.'[22] While the nation's military and political leaders saw this as a weakness, for a time it endeared shattered soldiers to the public who accorded them the same sympathy they showered on the sick and the wounded. In Australia this sympathy probably lingered for longer than it did in Britain, but with the approach of economic collapse in the thirties it diminished.

Because of censorship and the primitive propaganda then in place, people 'at home' had little concept of the real horrors of the war. They had been primed on the valorous military deeds of empire in which British arms triumphed over poorly armed, often primitive, adversaries. There was no artillery, poison gas, no trenches or the other panoply of this new 'world' war. Although the old image of chivalric deeds and conduct had been shaken briefly by the Boer War, the essentially rustic and heroic element of war had survived. New elements had also come of age. 'Two features of this industrial mode of warfare and its ideological and political framework have an important bearing on the social construction of shellshock—the "deskilled" nature of military work in the trenches and the ignorance on the part of the public back home in Britain [or Australia] about what life on the Western Front was actually like [and C.E.W Bean did little to disabuse them].'[23]

In the case of Australian civilians, distance interposed yet another filter to reality. London soon swarmed with the mental debris of the war making their way around town in the arms of nurses, bandaged, stammering uncontrollably or talking to themselves. Australia's cosmopolitan centres were spared that probably until late 1916. The population had little experience of any mass casualties as a result of the industrial age. 'The closest experience to trench warfare before winter 1914 in civilian society was to be found in the wreckage of a railway accident.'[24] This specific type of accident had set an important medical benchmark in Europe and the United States. The late nineteenth and early twentieth century industrial experience (railway accidents etc.) reflected 'a general view that some type of disturbance to the nervous system might be physically produced, without haemorrhage, either by temporary disablement of cells, or perhaps by the disruption of their connections.'[25] Unlike Britain and Germany, motor vehicle and industrial accidents were still relatively rare in a largely agrarian based Australia and so there was little exposure here.

However there were other parallels between life in Australia and the London metropolis. Since 1900 medical literature had increasingly advertised the presence of 'railway spine' and the reactions, physical and emotional, of industrial and transport accidents. And indeed there had been some spectacular rail accidents in Australia up to this time.[26] A booming industry in workers' compensation had begun in Britain, as it did in Germany, and was maturing as war broke out in 1914. The timing was unfortunate as many compensation doctors who worked for industry found themselves passing judgement on shell-shocked soldiers later in the war. They brought to their considerations their civilian experiences—particularly of fraud—and thus strengthened the link between shell shock and malingering. This too will be explored further. Frustratingly for the historian, the Provost Marshal's records of Australians arraigned for court martial, cowardice, self-inflicted wounds etc. were destroyed after the war.[27]

Shell shock as a mental phenomenon affected individuals, the evolution of psychology, the military, medicine, literature and society in a way rarely seen in modern history. It at once encompassed the deepest, most private recesses of the mind as well as the massive canvas that was the Great War. But it has never been dealt with in its entirety in any systematic way in Australian historiography. During the war, shell shock was not well understood and, paradoxically, despite the advances in knowledge since 1918, popular understanding of it within the collective memory of the Great War has not increased. 'Between the "strong" use of the term shell shock to describe the worst destructive effects of the war, and the "weak" use to describe an unpleasant emotional surprise of physical fatigue, there is a history of its transmission' through both British and Australian culture that continues to this day—a fragment of the fading collective memory.[28]

The numbers of afflicted soldiers were not inconsiderable. In 1914, 1,906 British troops presenting with behavioural disorders without physical cause were admitted to hospital. In 1915 the number grew to 20,327 or 9 per cent of battle casualties. By the end of the war '30,000 mental cases had been evacuated to England, and in 1922 some 50,000 men had been awarded war pensions on mental grounds alone.'[29] Corresponding figures for the AIF are difficult to obtain because of the lack of accurate statistics. For comparative purposes a total of 179,461 soldiers were listed as battle casualties (of all types) on the Western Front between 1916 and 1918. Of these 1,624 were classified as suffering from shell shock.[30] But this number *only* included soldiers who, in addition to being diagnosed as shell shocked, were also wounded. So the truer figure for all shell-shocked victims is likely to have been much higher. While the published statistics suggest a rate comparable to British casualty figures of about one per cent, the true number of mental casualties (including cases not formally reported at the time) is likely to be considerably more—possibly as high as eight per cent.[31]

The Australian military had hardly considered the matter of psychological casualties when the country answered Britain's call to arms in 1914. Later, some of the few practising 'psychologists' tried, in professional journals or in letters to the newspapers, to alert the army to the likelihood of such casualties and freely offered their services. As one of them wrote: 'The war may produce no new "psychoses", but it will doubtless bring us many unusual cases of neurasthenia, hysteria, phobias and obsessions of many kinds.'[32] He was right. By 1915 there were positive developments in managing this type of casualty, but these were generally restricted to Britain. The most visible example was 'the development of special hospitals...In the case of neurasthenia, the President of the Psycho-Medical Society wrote to the War Office in the first month of the war—before the problem of shell shock had attracted much attention—proposing an organization of hospitals for such cases. The first of these hospitals was opened in January 1915.'[33] Generally, in both countries, officialdom ignored both the psychologists' fears and their generosity. The medical fraternity too, wary of a long tradition of thriving quackery in mental health and jealous of its own professional prerogatives, continued to look askance at the new science and the 'alienists'—as the early psychologists were known.

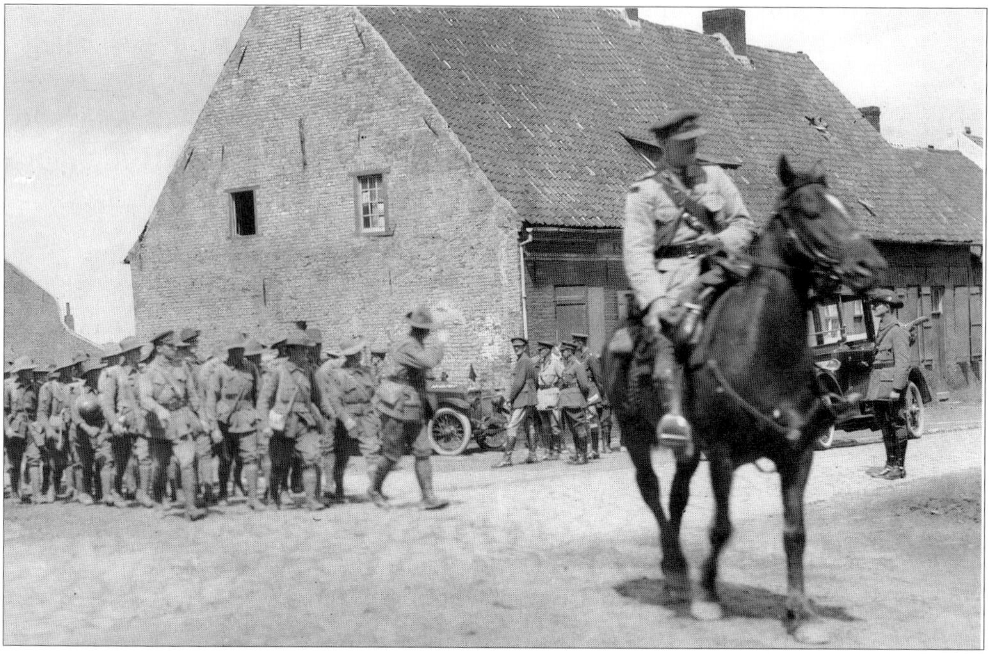

A photograph of Lieutenant-Colonel Arthur Butler at the head of the 3rd Field Ambulance at Hazebrouck, 10 August 1917. The author of Australia's official medical history, Butler did not absolve the shell-shocked from responsibility for their problems.
(AWM E04576 – image enhanced by the author)

For its part the military enshrined the epitome of the imperial male ideal. While the optimism of those first volunteers who flooded into recruiting centres might have been misplaced, there was no doubt in their minds that they could stick it and take whatever the barbaric Hun could hurl at them. But with the military and the system generally overwhelmed, many were fed into the system with often disastrous consequences both for the army and the individual. This is yet another part of the war modern-day Australians continue to overlook. Recruiting centres and overworked medical staff (with few guidelines to work by) were overrun and could scarcely do either their profession or the military justice by properly screening many recruits who should never have been allowed to don a uniform and who later would create a significant medical problem for the AIF and a burden on the taxpayer.[34] For his part, A.G. Butler was unambiguous in his opinion. The following paragraph, which appeared in a draft chapter of his official history, was never published: 'Both now and throughout the war, also, were men (in their sum amounting to many thousands) whose inclusion in the force, though unfit for service, was permitted by the examining officer at recruitment. It cannot too strongly be insisted that such action is almost as deserving of censure and even punishment as is concealment of disease.'[35]

Once in the thick of the fighting it wasn't long before 'weaknesses' started to show. In his analysis of the 1st Australian Division's casualties during the offensive at Pozières, Butler wrote that the casualty returns revealed 'the outstanding feature of the experience the emergence, as a major medical problem of the war (as it was to be of the peace), of the condition then known as "shell shock".'[36] Few Australians realise that, by early 1915, within days of the landing at Gallipoli, shell-shocked troops, real malingerers and others were being conveyed back to the hospitals and the other delights of Cairo to be treated or 'lost' to the army system for months. Some of these same men would be successful in applying for pensions on their return home, thereby adding another dimension to the confused situation in which genuine psychiatric casualties would find themselves on their return to civilian life.

Shell shock as a psychological phenomenon caught military medicine unawares, although the recent Russo–Japanese War had shown doctors a glimpse of what large-scale mechanised warfare might wreak upon the soldiery. Like most of the British dominions, Australia's contribution to World War One, while it was to have lasting effects at home, was relatively modest in the scale of things.[37] Once the bulk of the AIF left Egypt early in 1916, it became a small part in the massive allied war machine that was deployed along the Western Front. The Australian forces therefore relied for much of their logistical support and infrastructure on Britain and, to a lesser extent, its French ally. This was particularly the case for the treatment of mental illness. While the Australian Army Medical Corps (AAMC) had significant numbers of trained personnel both at the front and in numerous establishments scattered around Great Britain, it had very few specialists in the new field of psychology. Of these, most, as was the case in Britain, had been recruited from the civilian asylum system. But the asylums at home also had to be maintained with specialist staff who could not be readily released for the war effort.

Of necessity, therefore, the AIF had to rely on more established and certainly more numerous civilian and Royal Army Medical Corps (RAMC) staff to care for Australian 'mental cases'. Perhaps disingenuously, the official historian wrote that the Australian records do not contain sufficient material for a 'technical' examination of the problem of major psychoses in the war, in part because the AAMC had no responsibility for caring for psychological cases other than to repatriate them home.[38] How well they were managed is hard to gauge from this distance in time, as the vast and comprehensive collection of AIF medical records was destroyed in London shortly after the war. In wartime Britain, resources were few and many asylum doctors were soon pressed into army uniform and a number of military asylums such as Queen's Square, Netley, Harefield, and Napsbury were extended or established—almost all along strict class divisions between officers and Other Ranks. Not long into the war the profession itself became divided among various schools, of which Freud was only one protagonist. This dilution of resources into sometimes antagonistic methods of treating soldiers could only further delay or deny timely and appropriate treatment. Some men would never be relieved of their symptoms because of the multiplicity and sometimes incompatible courses of treatment available to doctors which they inflicted upon patients, even though some were in their care for only a few days. 'The Great War may have demonstrated beyond doubt that psychological agents can, by themselves, utterly disrupt the body's functions, but the lesson did nothing to mitigate the certainty that nervous breakdown unmanned men.'[39]

Editors, retired generals and politicians have never shied away from embroidering 'official' histories. The literature of the First World War was no stranger to censorship. What, for example, did Butler omit or edit? On the topic of death, in his published medical history he cited a private diary which agonised that only men who had themselves 'been through the mill' or who had their friends 'blown into hideous fragments, after hours of hell—*or who have seen him die a hideous death—or heard his squeals of agony and not been able to do anything for him* [deleted]...can have the proper treatment for dealing with men from the line who have got back for any reason.'[40] This was just one example of the many instances in which Butler believed the *lay* reader might be 'offended' or made 'squeamish' and therefore he deleted such unsavoury references. C. E. W. Bean was the journalist officially appointed to cover the war as it unfolded. He has been called 'the chief transmitter of the AIF stereotype on a national scale from the beginning of the war'.[41] Bean was not only Butler's senior editor, but had taken it upon himself to show the new nation of Australia in the best light to its own citizens and to the rest of the world. His was a finely articulated but flawed view of the war, as he 'sympathised with the world view of the senior officers' in whose inner circle he delighted.[42] The vehicle he chose was the corpus of painstakingly detailed notes kept between 1914 and 1918. The result assisted him in moulding the Anzac myth. Years after the First World War, Bean wrote of his history that its theme could be couched as an answer to the question of how did Australia, 'bred in complete peace...and the self discipline necessary for men who grapple with nature' react to what was 'the supreme test for fitness to exist?'[43] The Darwinian parallel is striking.

To Bean, who even in 1915 was starting to shape the malleable juvenile Australian abroad for popular consumption at home, shell-shocked men represented a profound threat and so were anathema to him. His was not an isolated position and the editor of the Canadian official medical history was blunt in his assessment. He identified shell shock as 'a manifestation of childishness and femininity. Against such there is no remedy.'[44] Perhaps in this assessment Canada's leading expert, C. K. Russel, had advised him. Russel had seen many patients who, although shell shocked, had either escaped heavy shelling or had been nowhere near the front.

After the fiasco of the failed Gallipoli campaign in which Australian, New Zealand, British and French troops took part, Bean set about publishing his *Anzac Book*, a panegyric to Australia's warrior sons. 'The Anzac Book is only a partial record of the way the Anzacs faced up to the challenge of Gallipoli.' It tells the story without the suffering, grief, bitterness or any of the human weaknesses that many of the soldiers wrote about. Although Bean was more than willing to include images and text that showed the difficulties faced by the men at Gallipoli, he rejected any poems or other material that depicted Australian losses in 'bitter or negative terms.'[45] These tended to surface in other media such as the wartime soldiers' magazine *Aussie*, over which Bean had no control. There is also no published Australian equivalent of British war poets like Sassoon, Brooke and Owen. The *Anzac Book* was Bean's creation, the first step in his memorialising of the AIF. 'The image of the Anzac it established was the product of his editorial activity.'[46] It remains with us.

But in this endeavour, as in his massive four-volume work of over 4,000 pages on the AIF's participation in the fighting on the Western Front, only one, volume III, mentions shell shock explicitly, and then there are only four short references.[47] This is not to suggest that Bean, himself a first-hand witness to many horrors of trench warfare, was not sympathetic to Australian soldiers. His published work, however, is less than even-handed when it comes to presenting the 'digger'. Praiseworthy as his efforts to commemorate them were, he did the war neurotic no great service. His field notes attest to many eyewitness accounts of shocked or neurotic soldiers and we will return to this in a later chapter. Interestingly too, Bean was careful to downplay any class differences within the AIF as this ran counter to the democratic image he was trying to nurture for Australia. As we shall see, social class—specifically the supposed differences between soldiers and officers—was at least a part of the perception by some of shell shock during the war. Bean also excluded manuscripts 'that contrasted the unequal comforts or sacrifices of officers and men, and included material which implied that the AIF had done away with class differences.'[48]

In summary, the shell shock crisis has been interpreted as a 'watershed' between an era when hereditarian, somatic and often inhumane approaches to care of the mentally disordered were the order of the day and a more enlightened 'postwar era of environmental, psychological and more humane attitudes.' Some see this type of interpretation as being 'deeply bound up with the mythology of the First World War.'[49] Shell shock specifically and war neuroses generally also had profound connotations for the individuals concerned. In a gender-biased observation A.G. Butler identified 'the chief war neuroses' as hysteria or the unconscious flight into disease which he found in war 'were even more diverse and bizarre than in the feminine type in peace.' The second neurosis was 'anxiety phobia' or worry.[50]

How did these 'phobias' affect soldiers on the battlefield and how were they managed or mismanaged in the field and further away from the fighting in hospitals and other centres of care? At the core of the military's attitude to the problem was what was seen as the soldiers' own failings. As the numbers of troops presenting with what appeared to be shell shock among otherwise sound men increased dramatically during 1917, the old excuse of weakness became less tenable. Answers had to be found to account for this aberration in male behaviour. 'Emotional control, the linchpin of male identity, was exactly what shell-shocked soldiers lacked. What would have been seen as unmanly behaviour bordering on cowardice or malingering was transformed when labelled "shell shock" so that it became more palatable.'[51] But shell shock remained very much an experience of the individual in much the same way that only a victim can experience a wound.

Endnotes

1 David Fromkin, *Europe's Last Summer: Why the World went to War in 1914*, Heinemann, London, 2004, p. 29.

2 The military psychological principles of 'proximity, immediacy and expectation' which later came to be widely used from World War II on, were apparently first used by the Russian Army in the Russo–Japanese War of 1905. E. Deane, *Shook Over Hell*, Harvard University Press, Mass., 1997, p. 31.

3 Eric Leed, *No Man's Land: Combat and Identity in World War One,* Cambridge, 1979, p. 164.

4 Stephen Garton, *The Cost of War: Australians Return*, Oxford, 1996, p. 145.

5 Joy Damousi, *The Labour of Loss: Mourning, Memory and Wartime*, Cambridge University Press, Melbourne, 1999, p. 96.

6 A. MacPhail, *Official History of the Canadian Forces in the Great War 1914–1919: the Medical Services*, Acland, Ottawa, 1925, p. 276.

7 Quoted in Robert Ahrenfeldt, *Psychiatry in the British Army in the Second World War*, Routledge & Keegan Paul, London, 1958, p. 10.

8 Janet Oppenheim, *Shattered Nerves: Doctors, Patients and Depression in Victorian England*, Oxford, 1991, p. 317.

9 R.J. Ørner, 'Post-Traumatic Stress Disorders and European War Veterans', *British Journal of Clinical Psychiatry*,' vol. 31, 1992, p. 387.

10 Garton, *The Cost of War*, p. 156.

11 Leese, *Shell Shock*, p. 157.

12 While the very succinctness and alliteration of 'shell shock' gave it a primacy in this war, such terminology is not unique. 'In each of the three wars in which Australia has been involved, an initial attempt was made to catch all of the psychopathology produced within one phrase. In the First War it was shell shock, in the Second War it was combat fatigue and in the Vietnam War it was post-traumatic stress disorder.' Robert Finlay-Jones, 'The Effect of War on Theory and Practice of Psychiatry in Australia', H. Attwood et al. (eds.), *Patients, Practitioners and Techniques*, 2nd National Conference in Medicine and Health in Australia, University of Melbourne, 1985, p. 46.

13 Feudtner, 'Minds the Dead Have Ravished', p. 399.

14 A. G. Butler, *Official History of the Australian Army Medical Services in War of 1914–1918, The Western Front,* vol. II, Australian War Memorial, Canberra, 1940, p. 99.

15 J. M. Winter, 'Shell-shock and the Cultural History of the Great War', *Journal of Contemporary History*, 35, 2000, p. 9.

16 T. A. Ross, *Lectures on War Neuroses*, Edward Arnold, London, 1941, p. 31.

17 Butler, *Official History*, vol. II, p. 72.

18 Leed, *No Man's Land*, p. 171.

19 The gender-specific association of hysteria is very evident in M. H. Downey's 'The Management and Treatment of Early Insanity', a paper read before the South Australian Branch of the British Medical Association and published in the *Australasian Medical Gazette*, 20 December 1911, p. 724.

20 Elaine Showalter, *The Female Malady: Women, Madness and English Culture 1830 –1980*, Pantheon, New York, 1985, p. 172.

21 Ibid., p. 172.

22 Leed, *No Man's Land*, p. 166.

23 Martin Stone, 'Shellshock and the Psychiatrists', in W. F. Bynum, R. Porter and M. Shepherd (eds.), *The Anatomy of Madness*, vol. II, London, 1985, p. 259.

24 Leese, *Shell Shock*, p. 15.

25 Harold Merskey, 'Shell-Shock', in H. Freeman and G. E. Berrios (eds.), *150 Years of British Psychiatry*, vol. I, London, 1991, p. 246.

26 For example, 43 people had been killed in a rail crash at Sunshine in Victoria in 1908.

27 Butler, *Official History*, vol. II, p. 90*n*. To the dismay of British commanders, there was no death penalty in the AIF. It was telling, however, that towards the end of the war when the strain was

becoming intolerable even for the most battle-hardened, 'the admission rate to prison for Australians was four times as high for soldiers of Canada and New Zealand, and eight times the rate of admissions for British soldiers.' Chris Pugsley, *The Face of Hell: New Zealanders and Military Discipline in the First World War*, Hodder & Stoughton, Auckland, 1991, p. 260.

28 Leese, *Shell Shock*, p. 161.

29 Dennis Winter, *Death's Men: Soldiers of the Great War*, Penguin, Melbourne, 1979, pp. 129–30.

30 A. G. Butler, *Problems and Services, The Australian Army Medical Services in the War of 1914-18*, vol. III, Australian War Memorial, Canberra, 1943, p. 912. Statistics throughout this book are used as indicative figures, rather than necessarily accurate raw data. Obtaining such figures is fraught with difficulty, as Butler and most other historians of the period recognised.

31 Butler suggests that for Gallipoli alone the percentage of men suffering from 'moral and mental disorders' was 2.3 per cent (see vol. III, p. 89) of all non-battle casualties. He also cites US and British authorities after the war suggesting that 65,000 ex-servicemen in the UK were in receipt of pensions on the grounds of shell shock, while 31.5 per cent of all ex-soldiers who had applied for war relief had some kind of neuropsychiatric disability (see vol. III, p. 129*n*).

32 W.E. Jones, 'Case of Shell Shock', *Medical Journal of Australia* (hereafter *MJA*), 4 March 1916, p. 203.

33 Roger Cooter, *Surgery and Society in Peace and War: Orthopaedics and the Organisation of Modern Medicine, 1880–1948*, London, 1993, p. 112.

34 For a more detailed analysis of the failures of recruit screening see Michael Tyquin, *Gallipoli: The Medical War*.

35 A.G. Butler, Medical History Drafts, Part I, vol. III, Chapter Two, AWM 44 16/4.

36 Butler, *Official History*, vol. II, p. 72.

37 See Appendix One at the end of this book.

38 Butler, *Official History*, vol. II, p.130.

39 Oppenheim, *Shattered Nerves*, p. 152.

40 Extract from an unidentified private diary in A.G. Butler's notes for the third volume of his official history. AWM 41 [658].

41 Lloyd Robson, 'The Australian Soldier: Formation of a Stereotype', in M. McKernan and M. Browne (eds.), *Australia: Two Centuries of War and Peace*, Australian War Memorial and Allen & Unwin, Canberra, 1988, p. 326. Although shell shock only affected a small percentage of the AIF, Butler's own notes for his aptly titled chapter 'The War-Damaged Soldier' has a mass of material that he collected for research and statistical purposes.

42 E. M. Andrews, *The Anzac Illusion: Anglo-Australian Relations during World War 1*, Cambridge University Press, Melbourne, 1993, pp. 214–15.

43 C. E. W. Bean, 'Our War History', *Bulletin*, 27 May 1942, p. 2.

44 MacPhail, *Official History of the Canadian Forces in the Great War 1914–1919: the Medical Services*, p. 278.

45 Alistair Thompson, *Anzac Memories: Living with the Legend*, Oxford, 1994, p. 68. One of these rejected poems is reproduced in the conclusion to this book.

46 D. Kent, 'The Anzac Book and the Anzac legend: C.E.W. Bean as Editor and Image Maker', *Historical Studies*, vol. 21, no. 84, April 1985, p. 387.

47 Not surprisingly, Butler, as the official medical historian, gave rather more space to the problem, with two chapters in the third volume dealing with war neuroses, while his other two volumes contain many references throughout.

48 Thompson, *Anzac Memories*, p. 68.

49 M. Thomson, 'Status, Manpower and Mental Fitness: Mental Deficiency in the First World War', in R. Cooter, M. Harrison and S. Sturdy (eds.), *War, Medicine and Modernity*, Stroud, 1999, p. 149.

50 Butler, *Official History*, vol. III, p. 18.

51 Feudtner, 'Minds the Dead Have Ravished', p. 403.

Chapter Three

Through a Glass Darkly

The phrase '...the war changed everything' often used to describe World War I can appear trite, but it could equally apply to the state of psychology in 1914.[1] Never again would the soldier be regarded *en masse* as an arm of war. The combatant now came to be seen as being vulnerable in ways rarely hinted at in Victorian and Wilhelmine depictions of war. 'Shell shock' was also the only medical term 'with a reference to war [although 'battle shock' was suggested at the time], but rejected during World War I in favour of standard psychiatric labels of disease...The rejection of the term shell shock early placed the emphasis on the weakness of the individual rather than the nature of war.'[2] The difficulty the military and the medical fraternity found in defining the problem, together with the perceived 'weakness' of the individual and his own responsibility for what the strain of battle did to him, are the main themes of this chapter.

Shell shock was a quintessential affliction of the individual. In modern society the image of the mentally damaged is at once both supremely personal and yet representative of that generation that initially flocked so readily to war. As we have already noted, it was a time of increasing sophistication in the application of industry and science to the ancient art of warfare. But this rapid development was unbalanced. 'Military psychology was in its infancy during the First World War, as physicians gradually appreciated that shell-shock, certain forms of trench fever and DAH [Disordered Action of the Heart, a major cause of invalidity in the Boer War] were functional disorders related to the stress of combat, whether actual or envisaged.'[3] While the science of killing people leapt ahead, the understanding of the mind subjected to such savagery trudged slowly in its wake.

This chapter will look firstly at the lesser known incidences of mental and other less easily labelled manifestations as they occurred at Gallipoli in 1915 and then scrutinise the AIF in France from 1916 to 1918. An attempt will then be made to survey the types of treatment that military medicine offered and their evolution during the war, together with the rationale behind their use. Finally we turn to the soldiers themselves to understand the impact of this war on individuals as well as looking at the views of others present on the battlefield or in the hospital system.

In 1914 Britain had deployed a small but professional army to France and the scale of psychological casualties was small. After all these men were highly trained and had been operating in fully functioning regiments and units, sometimes for years before. Kitchener's 'New Army', largely composed of civilian volunteers, was yet to make an impact. Australia's permanent soldiers were few indeed in 1914 and these consisted of a small cadre of full-time officers at command level. The vast majority of the first AIF were therefore untrained volunteers from all walks of life, but they were not all drawn from the youngest eligible age-group. What from 1915 would become a problem shared by both armies was a lack of appropriate medical and psychological screening during the recruiting process. Large numbers of men with serious forms of epilepsy and questionable mental stability, not to mention severe physical defects, managed to enlist. While there was no sophisticated scientific process then in place to assist the medical system to identify recruits with potential psychological issues, even a common-sense approach would have seen thousands denied entry to the army.[4]

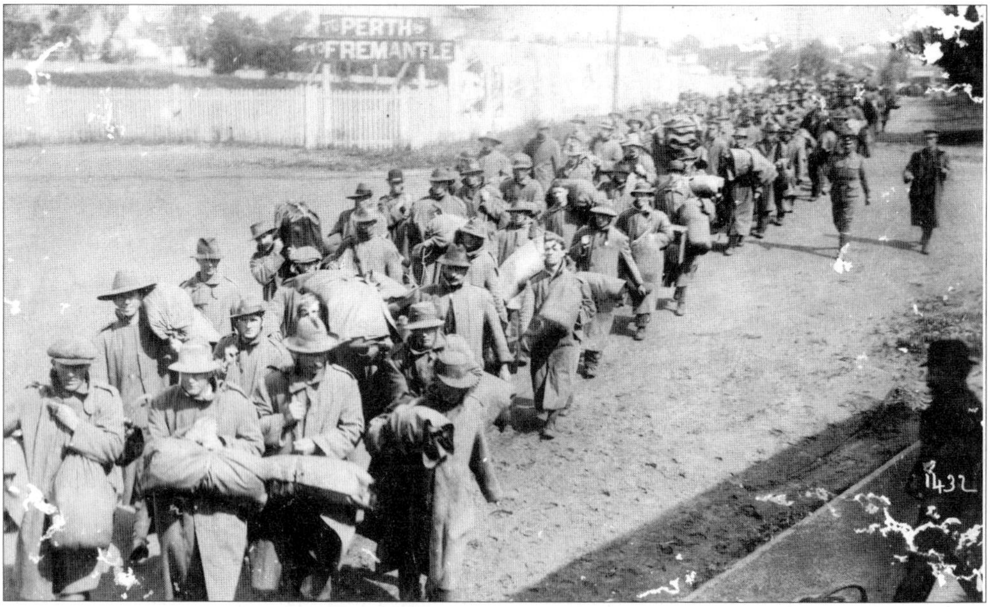

Recruits for the Australian Imperial Force with newly issued uniforms at Midland, Western Australia. For the first two years of the war, most recruits were poorly screened. False medical histories and outright lying did not help military medical authorities to identify those who did not meet the army's standards. (AWM P00088.014)

The official British military historian is disingenuous in his reasoning as to why there were so few psychologically unsuitable recruits. He explained that this 'could simply reflect that a very small number of mental defectives attempted to enlist.' He went on to state that while there was 'no clear evidence that a significant number did enlist, as such, the low rate can also be attributed to the limitations of mental testing.'[5] The Australian experience was that thousands of men who had enlisted were being sent home as early as 1915 due to medical and mental deficiencies.[6] Of these a large number would later try to claim war pensions. As one of Australia's senior medical consultants later noted of Gallipoli, 'Many cases of neurasthenia were boarded. Too many of them had neurasthenia before enlistment; there was often a definite history of treatment at hospitals in Australia for months before enlistment or inability to work at their usual occupation. Some of these looked upon Active Service as being likely to cure them and had even received such advice from their [civilian] medical attendant.'[7]

Unfortunately the rush of men young and old to the colours and the disposition of others to lie about their medical backgrounds, meant that even experienced doctors found the task of assessing recruits difficult. None of them had the time and some of them couldn't care. In Britain, as the war progressed, the drain of manpower caused by shell shock meant that 'concern over mental disorders centred on containment, rather than detection. Under such circumstances, there was little incentive to concentrate on exclusion of mental defectives from the Army.'[8] By contrast, in Australia the AAMC constantly fought a rearguard action against attempts by the government (especially in 1917 when its conscription referendum failed) to lower physical entry standards for recruiting to the AIF. Looking back on this situation from 1937, the Repatriation Commission's senior medical officer would recall that 'except in cases of extreme mental deficiency, selection for enlistment' would not inoculate a man 'against the chance of future admission to a mental hospital.' He was of the firm belief that 'an undue proportion of the vagrant and mentally unstable [note the combination] were, at one time or another during the war, enlisted...'[9] So, at the outbreak of war, we have a pool of men in the army who were psychotic, neurotic or borderline psychiatric cases before they had even donned a uniform. We also have the entrenched belief by many in both the military and the medical service that war-related neurosis was an hereditary issue. The approach to, and management of, shell shock would become their common battleground.

What was the scale of the problem faced by the army and its medical services? To help us position the problem within the period 1915–1918 we must resort to somewhat flawed statistical data to make detailed analysis and comparison possible.[10] Judicious use of these figures will lend some perspective while providing an idea of the magnitude of the problems not only for the military but also for its medical services. At first, in 1914, there was only a trickle of psychological casualties, no more perhaps than would be expected. 'In an official report written in December 1914, it is stated that 7 to 10 per cent of all officers, and 3 to 4 per cent of men admitted to hospitals in Boulogne were sent home suffering from the effects of nervous and mental shock, due to strain, stress and exhaustion.'[11] But as the war dragged on, the numbers of mentally afflicted soldiers grew.

At Gallipoli during 1915 British hospital admissions (many of whom were subsequently discharged that year) totalled 841 Other Ranks and 138 officers for neurasthenia, shell shock, and hysteria, while 2 officers and 72 Other Ranks were treated for 'mental diseases'.[12] Comparable figures for Australian troops at Gallipoli are difficult to ascertain but, according to Butler, there was a 'large evacuation from psycho-somatic breakdown' from Gallipoli.[13] In France, because of the significantly larger number of troops, the intensity of the fighting, and its long duration, the number of psychological casualties was correspondingly higher. 'From September 1914 to December 1917 the total British cases of shell shock reported totalled 26,938.'[14] The problem in the British Expeditionary Force (BEF) did not become acute until July 1917, during the blood-bath of the Somme (before that time shell shock cases were noticeably inconspicuous according to A.G. Butler) and this pattern was the same for British and Australian 'mental' casualties in France.

Reported Psychological Casualties—Britain and Australia[15]

British (excluding dominions):		Australian Imperial Force:
1914	9	-
1915	1,387	-
1916	20,089*	613
1917	7,048	895
1918	N/A	116
Total:	28,533	1,624

[*Mainly incurred in the second half of 1916]

The overall picture for Australian soldiers was that from the time the first convoy of invalids returned from England to Australia on 6 October 1915 until 24 August 1918 when the last convoy left, 19,254 sick and wounded casualties were sent home. Under 'Nervous Cases' these included 878 men suffering from shell shock, 1,433 with 'Disordered Action of the Heart' (DAH), 545 with neurasthenia and 308 epileptics, while 60 soldiers were classified as 'nervous' and a further 139 as 'mental' cases.[16]

As we have observed not all casualties had suffered the horrors of trench warfare. Of those diagnosed as suffering from 'Disorders of the Mind' and repatriated home, those with 'Front Line service' totalled 4,984 (or 8.47 per cent) of invalids with front line service, while those who had never been at the front accounted for 571 (3.96 per cent) of the 43,465 men who had not seen active service. 'The annual rate (per 1,000) of the AIF (on the Western Front only)' so classified totalled 16.96 per cent.[17] However the statistics for both the Australian and British armies should be treated with caution.

The figures also differ between sources, as another officer who wrote to Butler after the war gave these estimates: 'By the end of the war 849 men had been invalided to Australia for "mental trouble", 588 with service and 261 with "no service". Of the deaths of such men during the war, 112 were from self-inflicted wounds and 12 from "insanity"; 2 specified as "GPI" [General Paralysis of Insane]; while 29 men died from alcoholism.'[18] As the compilers of these statistics themselves admitted, they present formidable difficulties of interpretation. 'First, there was diagnostic confusion: hysterical symptoms were often mistaken for signs of organic disease and these cases ended up in the medical wards of base hospitals...Second, medical officers on the line were often reluctant to give a psychiatric diagnosis because of the stigma attached, preferring to use the label "sick" or "debility."'[19]

The central place of diagnosis or misdiagnosis in arriving at accurate figures for psychiatric casualties from the battlefield should not be underestimated. A further complication was the diversity and method of presentation of various signs and symptoms of shell shock. The waters of divination were further muddied by two other medical phenomena in vogue at the time—'Disordered Action of the Heart' (DAH) and 'Effort Syndrome'. In the case of Australian RMOs there is sufficient anecdotal evidence to suggest that many gave their patients the benefit of the doubt and diagnosed them with something other than 'mental' to avoid the stigma attached to such a label.

It Would Make the Strongest Man Quail

Shell shock was an omnibus term which encompassed the full gamut of neuroses or mental illnesses characterised by irrational or depressive thought, or behaviour linked (in most, but not all cases) to direct battlefield experience. It did not,

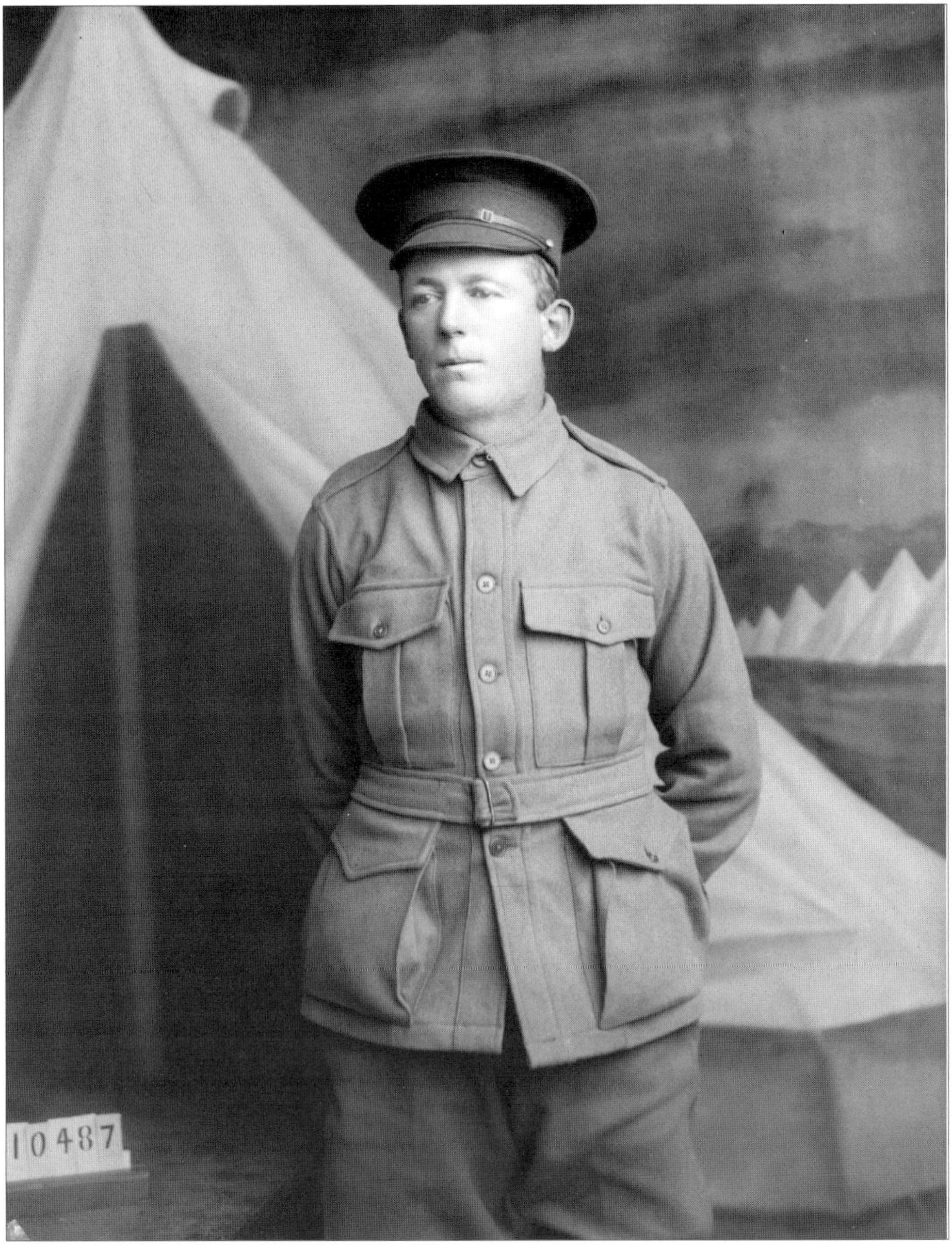

Private Alfred Kirkwood of the 7th Battalion was twice gassed in the trenches and suffered shell shock on the second occasion. Numbers of these men had been wounded or concussed not once, but several times, but they still managed to return to the trenches. Broadmeadows training camp, Melbourne, September 1916.
(AWM DA0487)

however, include psychoses or severe mental derangement which were relatively few during the war, although their incidence would rise during the 1920s. But what it all meant for the war effort and for medicine generally was as yet unknown. The other important element in the subsequent treatment and scientific debate was the place of the observer. This had been noted before the war as one Australian doctor (W. Beattie-Smith, New South Wales Inspector General of the Insane) put it in 1911: 'Up to the present we have been content to group the causative factors of insanity under general headings, and these general headings are largely filled up according to the personal *bias* of the particular recorder.'[20] The military was becoming increasingly nervous that this problem might be a drain on manpower, while military medicine was still unsure, although it continued to meet its obligation to return sick and wounded men to the front when fit again—as was its mandate. As there were various manifestations of shell shock, 'their meaning was open to dispute.'[21]

Accurate diagnosis and understanding of the aetiology, or how shell shock occurred, was not helped by the primitive scientific and medical knowledge at the time. This ignorance was compounded by the general disorientation caused by the war on all participants—at home and on the front. The old divisions of sanity and madness now seemed inadequate and could not explain how 'the individual [fitted] into the larger machine, and what should be done when he breaks down? Modern society had produced this illness and then framed it in modern garb, redefining individuality and responsibility in the process.'[22] But it was different closer to events. Butler, like his mentor and editor, Charles Bean, considered psychiatric casualties to be primarily 'moral and mental disorders'.[23] However he did recognise the unpreparedness of the medical profession generally to cope with the numbers of soldiers who presented with mental health problems during the war.[24] This was certainly the experience of the Australian Army Medical Corps.

In 1914 and 1915, men who were found staggering disoriented from bombed or collapsed trenches, but who exhibited no obvious signs of external wounds, were believed to have been simply concussed. In 1916 Australian medical officers (who had seen similar cases at Gallipoli) noted the increasingly common phenomenon at first hand. They believed that, while there were large numbers of so-called 'shell shock' cases, most men were simply suffering from exhaustion. Owing to the intensity of the bombardment and the pulverised nature of the soil, men were continually being buried and being dug out by their companions. 'After one such experience a man was buried and exhausted and they were fortunate who did not have that unpleasant experience. When it was repeated, as it often was several times, even the strongest collapsed and had to be evacuated.'[25] As the war along the Western Front intensified, the incidence of men being blown up and buried three or more times became commonplace. Their stoicism is remarkable from this distance in time and by no means did all of them present with neuroses.

'It was evident that some shell shock victims displayed symptoms akin to the condition known to doctors as "hysteria". Others appeared to be suffering from severe forms of "neurasthenia". These were two conditions, which at the time were held in low medical esteem.' Again the implications of moral weakness and associations of femininity are strong. Against this background and in view of their pre-1914 approach to hysteria and neurasthenia, it was 'unsurprising that the "experts" back home in the hospitals in the UK rapidly came up with an "organic" interpretation of shell shock's pathology.'[26] In other words the cause was believed to be physical and, therefore, the result also had to be physical even though the mechanism of injury was little understood. Learned articles appeared about microscopic lesions in the brain and the shaking of neurones. It was perhaps understandable that science should follow this path because to admit that men—particularly soldiers—could be suffering from the archetypal 'emotional' condition of hysteria would be to break a military taboo. At this phase of the war casualties included both officers and professional soldiers, so the later view of a moral problem or an inherent weakness within the casualty was not then raised. To do so would by implication have been to admit a national flaw which, in wartime, would have been disastrous to morale while offering the Germans a propaganda opportunity.

The prevailing perception at the time is illustrated in this statement from an Australian medical officer, Major A.W. Campbell. He reflected a popular bias in his description of what was believed at first to cause the problem, noting the most common signs and symptoms of the casualty:

> Almost without exception the subjects were young and *obviously* [emphasis added] neurotic...In most the cause was a severe shock, such as a shell explosion close at hand, lifting them into the air and burying them with debris, and perhaps, but not necessarily, rendering them unconscious. Cases of speech affection, aphonia, anarthria, mutism, or stammering were most frequent.[27]

The other aspect to many medical cases was the frequency with which men were blown up. This is hardly surprising in some parts of the front where huge amounts of high explosive were used by both sides. It has been estimated that, in one battle on the Somme, the British 'threw approximately 400,000 shells weighing about 7.5 million pounds into not more than 18,000 yards of enemy trench' in only two days. [28] How did these statistics translate to the soldiers in the field? Tasmanian Archie Barwick, a non-commissioned officer in C Company of the 1st Battalion confided in his diary:

> When you are in a bombardment, it makes you realise how small and puny a man's strength is when he is face to face with these powerful and terrible weapons of man's brain. It would make the strongest man quail for you are so helpless against it. You can only crouch down and wait for the worst, every minute you are expecting to be blown to pieces.[29]

It was the sense of helplessness and the fear of mutilation that were key factors in war neuroses on the Western Front. The miracle is that so many survived—mad or otherwise.

The following excerpts are from typical case notes on several psychological casualties, although the identities of the men are disguised.[30] They are, each in their own right, eloquent portraits of the fragility of the human mind under inhuman strain. Contrary to Major Campbell's view, all were healthy men prior to their injuries and, with one exception, they had no previous history of psychological problems.

Private W, a labourer, enlisted early in 1915 and was bombed at Messines on 20 September 1917 and admitted to hospital with shell shock. 'Suffers from continued headaches—giddy at times, slight insomnia, is neurasthenic and debilitated. Hearing impaired—great loss of energy. Blown up at least twice.'[31] Private B, a 26-year-old former clerk and now in the 3rd Battalion, had been in the AIF just under a year when he became a casualty late in 1917. 'Patient was wounded by a shell splinter while in support line...He was coming out when he was blown up a second time and badly concussed.' Five months later he still had 'great difficulty in articulation on account of stammering which has been persistent since concussion, is nervous and highly excitable and tremulous. Can only speak in a weak, low voice, chiefly does not attempt to answer orally, writes his answers down. Not considered permanently disabled, but minimum time for treatment, 7 months.'[32] Twenty-four-year-old Private M, who had also enlisted in 1915, was admitted to hospital diagnosed with shell shock after being hit by a shell at Bullecourt in May 1917. By January the following year he was described as 'a complete nervous wreck. Staring wildly, eyes bulging with tremors on any sharp or unusual sounds. Speech hesitating. Memory at times seems to [desert] him.

Sleeps badly, waking at intervals terrified.'[33] Private A was unlucky enough to be in charge of a water carrying party when they took shelter from an artillery barrage in a concrete pillbox. Unfortunately it was struck by a direct hit, buried by debris and then blown sky high. The victim was later described as 'very shaky, constant tremor of head, arms etc. Stuttering speech, sweating headaches.'[34] Early in 1918 Private L was blown up by a shell and spent eleven months in hospital. He complained to his doctors of 'shakiness and pains over heart and shortness of breath. Sometimes feels faint and cannot sleep but is improving.'[35]

The emergence of neuroses early in the war called for a rethinking of the way medicine regarded mental illness. Psychology was still finding its feet in 1914 and was yet to consolidate a position in the medical sciences at least as a profession in its own right. It was widely regarded among the establishment with suspicion, bordering in some cases on accusations of quackery. Its practitioners, known as 'alienists', also used a lexicon not widely understood by either physicians or surgeons, the same men who would become officers in the AAMC and RAMC. 'The medical officer at the front had no knowledge of the jargon in which the problem was being discussed.'[36] Eventually, as the war dragged on, a certain conformity emerged. 'For all the parties concerned hysteria and neurasthenia formed the chief categories in which psychologically wounded servicemen were classified.'[37]

Lieutenant-Colonel W.W. Hearne of the 2nd Australian Field Ambulance reported that between 22 July and 16 August 1916, a total of 7,183 casualties (excluding sick) passed though his unit. Of 79 officers, ten were 'shell-shocked' or about 12 per cent of the whole. Some 1,610 or approximately 22 per cent of Other Ranks were shell shocked. Most of these were sent to a Corps rest station that had been established during this period of fighting. Hearne concluded that many of these cases 'would be more appropriately described as physical or nervous exhaustion and they should be classified as sick rather than wounded.'[38] He was right in his assessment and there is no doubt that, early in the war, many men who were simply overworked or fatigued, were lost to the war effort through misdiagnosis. They were evacuated to the rear or to 'Blighty' and often back to Australia for discharge to become a medical puzzle for the postwar authorities.

The difficulty in accurate diagnosis implied here and the subsequent inclination of most AAMC officers to give these casualties the benefit of the doubt was still in evidence as late as August 1918. Charles Bean, writing of the RMO of the 58th Battalion, described a scene in which a medical officer told him of a good number of complaints which he could not easily diagnose. In Bean's presence the doctor then went outside his regimental aid post and spoke with some of the men. 'One chap was groaning whenever he was spoken to; the doctor spoke to him sharply, but he only groaned still.' Another man appeared, by Bean's own admission to have shell shock, but when the major asked the casualty if he felt better he said that he did, sufficiently well for him to return to the line. There were three or four other complaints at this outpost —all much of the same sort. Bean went on to write that he remembered seeing a few cases even on Gallipoli. The medical major was clearly sympathetic to the men and could 'hardly blame them.' According to Bean's notes 'a doctor's position is very different in these cases.' The major ended up sending all these men to the rear, 'but ordered notes to be kept of all cases' as per the Deputy Director of Medical Service's recent instructions to the Army.'[39]

Medical science was soon being pressed for answers and these were made hesitatingly and were slow in coming. This piece, from H. Wiltshire, a British doctor in 1916, represents one school of thought at the time and is quoted at length as it encompasses a number of the issues that will be discussed further. 'At the present time...the etiology [sic] of "shell-shock" is buried in confusion, owing to three main difficulties, namely: 1. Bad terminology...2. Dubious clinical histories...3. Rapid changes in clinical condition...' In looking at possible 'psychic causes', he suggested 'gradual psychic exhaustion from continued psychic strain', as 'a cause of neurosis per se.' Wiltshire also proposed that in 'most cases of shell shock the immediate cause of the nerve collapse is to be found in some sudden psychic shock. The various events which may produce such sudden shock are (1) horrible sights, (2) losses, (3) fright from an explosion, or (4) sounds [often a combination of these].' [40]

In the following year the authoritative *Medical Annual* could only describe shell shock as a term 'loosely used to describe a variety of conditions'.[41] Science remained baffled. Butler, too, sketched out a chronology of 'shell shock' or 'a sequence of the neurotic constitution' thus: mental conflict; the anxiety state; moral and mental and perhaps a physical shock; stupor; confusion and amnesia; and psycho-neuroses.[42] However a modern-day scholar has provided a comprehensive list of how a shell-shocked soldier might present:

> The symptoms associated with 'shell shock' were varied, from vague anxiety, depression, startle reactions, an inability to concentrate one's thoughts, loss of memory, insomnia, nightmares, intense fear, 'trotting heart', and panic attacks to uncontrollable shaking, aphonia, mutism, hysterical blindness, amnesia, partial or total paralysis, and hysterical fits, in which the subject might scream and blindly thrash about in depression.[43]

Towards the end of 1916 the British military decided to divide all cases diagnosed in the field as shell shock into two categories. The first was to be called 'Shell Concussion' and included 'those cases showing actual signs and symptoms of concussion of the brain or spinal cord of a severe nature', i.e. injuries consistent with the consequences of high explosive shells. The second category was now to be called 'Nervous Shock'. This would include all other cases that could be grouped under the term 'inability to stand shell fire'. Soldiers within the first category were to be evacuated 'wounded' in the usual way, while the latter would be classified as 'sick' and directed to special casualty clearing stations where, after investigation, 'a case may be diagnosed "shell shock".'[44]

We have mentioned two other little-understood conditions that were often included in diagnoses, treatment and discussion of genuine war neuroses. A leading Australian medical officer, Lieutenant-Colonel J. W. Springthorpe, put the case succinctly when he wrote about the 'Effort Syndrome'—also known as Da Costa Syndrome, after an American Civil War doctor's observations. He thought that 'the physiological and the psychological are so mixed up that their dissociation and analysis lead only to a clinical phantasy [sic] and thus to a field of therapeusis not proper to the Freudian nor to the neo-cardiologist, nor yet to the physiotherapist.'[45] But what was first thought to be a physiological problem was later included in the still-unclear understanding of war neuroses. Butler concluded that, in Effort Syndrome patients, 'we may infer that any distress experienced during or shortly after physical exertion is not due to any fundamental weakness of the *cardiovascular* system. Rather it is an indication of abnormal *nervous* reaction.'[46] In a pamphlet written for army doctors in the Second World War, the Effort, or Da Costa, Syndrome was described as commencing as an anxiety state. Later, the emotional element would disappear, being 'converted' into a physical manifestation as the emotional symptoms waned when the unconscious provided an adequate face-saving mechanism. 'There seems no doubt that the vast majority of these should be treated as a mere variant of the fear complex.'[47] The second condition had been identified in the Boer War. Disordered Action of the Heart (DAH) was attributed to soldiers' experiencing fatigue after battle or long marches. Those affected presented with a weak but rapid pulse (tachycardia), lack of breath, exhaustion and lapses of concentration.

These two 'conditions' illustrated the poorly understood relationship between physical and physiological factors. An AAMC officer, Lieutenant-Colonel D. McWhae, wrote that DAH eventually 'proved one of the most clinically obscure among the "medical" conditions causing disablement and one of the most difficult to deal with.' The term, banned on 29 May 1918, was replaced by the diagnosis

'Effort Syndrome'—'in view of the fact that "there was no evidence that the condition was cardiac in origin."'[48] Unfortunately this did not help matters, and so accurate identification of war neurosis was made harder by the continued suspicion of DAH in the minds of doctors. Writing in 1940 a clinician noted that cardiovascular diseases were the second largest cause of illness in the British Army in World War I. He correctly concluded that 'Effort Syndrome' was nothing more than a collection of signs and symptoms—which often included breathlessness, exhaustion and tremors—rather than a disease in itself.[49]

Malingering—Real or Sham?

Contrary to popular belief not every digger who set foot in Egypt, Gallipoli, France or Belgium was a hero. Any serious Australian study on the subject of malingering is bedevilled by a lack of source material as Butler himself had to concede. He admitted that, despite the interest in the subject, no statistics had been compiled to reflect what he called 'the unconscious escape into disease' (hysteria), the 'conscious escape into disease' (malingering), and 'the escape' into self-inflicted wounds and 'the escape into death' (suicide).'[50] The same held true for breaches of discipline including soldiers going absent without leave. C.E.W. Bean also ignored these same 'weaknesses'. There is little doubt that, in 1915, some soldiers were in Egypt for what they could get out of it. Others, once the scent of battle reached their nostrils, changed their minds, while some men simply fled as the opportunity arose.

Mention has been made of poor screening processes; we will now examine their implications for the AIF and its medical services in the Mediterranean. One doctor had little sympathy for these flighty fighters:

> Before our arrival in Egypt malingerers in the force [AIF] who, having enjoyed a holiday trip to Egypt, wanted to go home again, suddenly discovered that they were blind or deaf. For a time the [outpatient's] department was fairly busy detecting the wiles of these men. When they discovered, however, that they would be subjected to expert examination, sight and hearing soon returned. A number of devices were resorted to in order to detect the fraud—ie. the use of faradisation [electric shocks], blind-folding and the like—and it was rarely that the imposter escaped.[51]

We have alluded to the connection between mental disorders and the fashionable early twentieth century idea that these conditions posed 'moral' questions or revealed moral weaknesses. Suspicions were usually linked to one of two social shortcomings. The first was the hereditary aspect of mental illness, which was considered a social infirmity. A very important element in the bio-medical thought of that time was the concept that anyone who became a casualty of shell shock and its associated signs and symptoms must have been more or less predisposed to it. 'A person's hereditary temperament was meant to play a large role in his being predetermined in this way.'[52] Medical practitioners, sure of their own genetic or aesthetic superiority, sometimes linked appearance with IQ. Private C of the 4th Battalion, a former blacksmith who had enlisted in January 1915, suffered shell shock and spent months in various hospitals in the UK. Unflattering portraits of such men, such as that reproduced here, are not unusual to find in doctors' notes, but they would probably be absent from any description of an officer suffering from the same condition. 'Patient has a somewhat *degenerate appearance, large ears, facial asymmetry...facile manner.*'[53] Another example was Private G, suffering from 'melancholia' or depression, from his experiences in France in August 1916. The medical officer treating him wrote that he 'was found wandering about by the Military Field Police in a confused state. Memory stated to be complete blank. He was violent to the guard...Remembers leaving Australia and going to Egypt and France.' He observed his patient to be '*Intensely dull and stupid.* Sits quietly uninterested in his environment...tremors and twitching.'[54] Observations such as these reveal as much about the doctor as they do about the patient.

The second social shortcoming was the belief that malingering, or even desertion from the trenches, was the action of the morally weak. In addition to their other problems, soldiers with neuroses were further weighed down by these perceptions of them as unreliable in the face of fire and as being likely cowards. These same cultural attitudes often coloured the medical treatment these men subsequently received.

Official histories of war usually paint an ideal picture, given that they are often an extension of government propaganda, albeit it after the event. They are edited, sanitised and often heavily censored despite the claims of their respective editors. Mistakes in war are blamed on others or put down to serendipity, blemishes are erased from the national character, shortcomings carefully disguised. Official histories are then a sort of giant marketing exercise in which countries put the best face on what was usually a chronicle of trial and error, false starts, bad planning or simply incompetence on the battlefield. The British and Australian histories were of this mould. According to the British, 'true malingering was very rare and could only be definitely proven in very few cases'[55] although, in a surprisingly sympathetic vein it recognised that a 'slightly confused individual, or a patient with severe anxiety neurosis, or even a dispirited, exhausted soldier may fail to meet the demands of military discipline, and in this may bring himself into a position of utmost seriousness.'[56] It went on to suggest that a few cases of desertion (a capital crime in the British Army) may have been caused by mental illness, including epilepsy, delusional insanity and dementia.[57] By then of course it was too late for the men who had been shot by a firing squad. The Australian case is bedevilled by a lack of extant source material. While C.E.W. Bean does mention episodes of desertion and ill-discipline in several of his volumes on the AIF in France, there is little statistical data.[58]

The medical aspect further muddied the waters for doctors at the front whose duty was to diagnose these men, a responsibility that could take on a judicial aspect. 'There was a general recognition on the part of medical officers that in administering the ambiguities of neurosis and in judging the "legitimacy" of the symptom, they had assumed certain judicial and political functions.'[59] This role never sat well with most medical officers and their discomfort is evident in a number of doctors' diaries and letters. This was certainly the case where self-inflicted wounds were suspected. 'There can be no doubt that for many doctors during the First World War the experience of dealing with malingerers compounded an already existing tension in the performance of their duty...To suspect a soldier of malingering was to enter into a relationship which was essentially adversarial.'[60] However there is certainly enough evidence to suggest that malingering was practised in the AIF and often doctors identified it for what it was.

While malingering and self-inflicted wounds have long been part of war, both elements have largely been forgotten in Australia in its commemorations of World War I. While we celebrate ingenuity in battle, this rarely extends to less heroic practices, no matter what desperation drew some soldiers to them. At Gallipoli it was a cause for scandal to some commanders. Brigadier Sinclair-MacLagan chided one of his battalion commanders that the incidence of self-inflicted injuries from gunshot wounds by men in his unit 'shows a lack of discipline and supervision by officers and NCOs which you must take steps to rectify without delay.' He recommended that all the men's rifles be examined by an officer and 'on every occasion of a change from firing line to support or reserves [lines], and vice-versa.'[61] In France conditions were less forgiving. A 29-year-old private of the 28th Battalion who had enlisted in August 1915 sailed full of expectation to England—where he stayed. At Weymouth Training Camp in England 'he got depressed and attempted suicide by cutting his throat because he did not get to the firing line.' He was in hospital one month, then in Netley Hospital four days and sent to a mental hospital in Scotland for six months.[62]

Not all neuroses were the result of being blown up or buried by high explosive. A 26-year-old private of the 41st Battalion who had enlisted early in 1915 was later diagnosed with 'Melancholia' or depression. He had been admitted to a field ambulance in France with a slight gunshot wound. Shortly after it was reported that for several day he had been 'strangely silent and preoccupied, refuses to answer questions, threatens suicide.' He was then transferred to a hospital and complained that his fellow patients were persecuting him. He admitted 'having opened a razor with suicidal intent.' The man was described as being listless, depressed and 'somewhat hopeless'. He was then admitted to D Block, Netley Hospital, in July 1918 where he 'hears people talking about him and says unpleasant things. Solitary and self-centred.' After a few weeks he was moved to the Lord Derby War Hospital before being returned to Australia almost a year later. This man had 'a previous history of mental breakdown as a fourteen-year old.' What was the diagnosis? His clinical notes stated he had a 'hereditary predisposition aggravated by active service and stress of campaign.'[63]

Those addicted to alcohol also wasted much of the army's time as can be shown in the case of a 36-year-old former station hand. Enlisting in August 1914 and sailing to Egypt with the First AIF, he was sent to the Special Hospital Abbassia, Cairo in October 1916. Diagnosed with 'Alcoholic Insanity' he was 'suspicious and the subject of nocturnal hallucinations, voices, animals etc. Cause: Intemperance.' He was consequently discharged to Australia.[64]

In recording total AIF shell shock casualties for France and Flanders during the war as 1,624 soldiers, there were also '700 *reported* [emphasis added] cases of "self-inflicted wounds."'[65] Self-inflicted wounds were the most obvious form of self-injury, but there were other, less obvious tricks such as adding egg whites to urine to mimic kidney disease, chewing cordite to cause an irregular heartbeat, or digesting picric acid to imitate jaundice.[66] This practice and the frequency with which men resorted to it received scant mention in Australian military histories then or since. Malingering did exist, but probably not to the extent some senior army officers liked to believe.

Of course Australian soldiers were not slow to pick up on the latest fads for getting out of the trenches, and sometimes their motives could be construed as altruistic. In a SECRET memorandum dated 17 May 1918, Colonel D. M. McWhae, an Assistant Director of Medical Services within the AIF who was based in Britain, forwarded to his headquarters a strange letter. The correspondence was from a Private W. Naughton, 25th Battalion, written in France on 29 April 1917 to his brother L.B. Naughton who was then in a training battalion. Unfortunately the censor had intercepted it.

> ...I'm writing to let you know of a stunt for getting home. You'll know by the writing who it comes from. All you want is a piece of toilet soap, a lighted candle and a good fire. Rub soap round the joints of your foot, a good dose, not in a lather then bandage it up with a very thin rag. Drop hot candle grease on where the soap is and let it settle. Then hold your foot to the [fire]. Do this for two nights and if my information is correct you ought to go home...This stunt is for you only. I'm going you pull it on toot sweet. I don't like to think I'm a squib but frig em I've done enough for the two of us...Hope to gee this letter gets through ok and no one meddles with it. I think I can kid the Lieut. to sign it without reading it.
>
> P.S. Do you know about the iodine cigarette—make a fag and drop six or seven drops of iodine on the 'bacca and roll it up. You will then have a bad heart [tachycardia] and a high temperature. Smoke the fag for an hour or so before going on sick parade.[67]

Until this time various senior medical officers had a suspicion, but no evidence, that soldiers adulterating their cigarettes with iodine were causing DAH. Other commentators looked for explanations for unsoldierly conduct in racial stereotypes. The Canadian official medical historian, for example, wrote that at 'the battle of Ypres in 1915 the practice [of self-inflicted wounds] was observed among the coloured troops.' He then raised the crucial dilemma posed for medical officers: 'Under cover of these vague and mysterious symptoms the malingerer found refuge, and impressed a stigma upon those who were suffering from a real malady. The medical officer was bewildered in his attempt to hold the balance between injustice to the individual and disregard for the needs of the service.'[68] Even so, malingering was an ever-present threat to the discipline of the AIF as it was across the Western Front and on both sides.

There were, however, circumstances in which medical officers would have fallen back on experience and their own feelings before making a hasty diagnosis. Private Roy Ramsay, a member of the 3rd Australian Field Ambulance, wrote of the atmosphere at Pozières. There, the aid posts and dressing stations to the rear of the front line were starting to fill with soldiers presenting with various battle injuries. Among these was a sprinkling of soldiers who 'were shaking like a leaf as a result of the bombardment and one runner even shot himself rather than go back up the line.' He went on to write that several soldiers were 'refusing to go back and would have been happy to be court-martialled and sent back to Australia.'[69] Had Ramsay been closer to the forward trenches he would have been even more dismayed by the scenes there. Corporal Archie Barwick again: 'As the ground heaved under the frightful bombardment any amount of men were driven stark staring mad and more than one of them rushed out of the trenches towards the Germans, any amount of them could be seen crying and sobbing like children, their nerves completely gone. How on earth anyone could stand it God alone knows. We were nearly all in a state of silliness and half-dazed.'[70]

Australian front line medical units 'picked up' most of these men later and RMOs, many of them close to the same bombardments, were in no position to doubt the veracity of the symptoms of these men. Reporting on a speech made by Major A.W. Campbell in 1916, in which he recounted his experiences abroad, the *Medical Journal of Australia* noted that shell-shocked patients Campbell had seen 'included many exaggerators, but very few malingerers.'[71] This is probably typical of officers' experiences within the AAMC generally.

As the war progressed and 'dramatic new medical knowledge' was incorporated into military medicine, 'the relativity between psychological illness and malingering remained ambiguous.'[72] However the place of malingering in the official mind had been cemented much earlier in the war. Commenting on a rather sensational case in Melbourne towards the close of 1915 the *Medical Journal of Australia* left its subscribers in no doubt where it stood on the issue. The case concerned a soldier who had been kicked by a horse in Egypt and repatriated to Australia. He subsequently alleged that the treating doctor had applied electric currents to his face to determine the veracity of his complaint. The soldier then fled to the house of a local parliamentarian where he sought sanctuary. He was forcibly removed and returned to hospital. The victim then took the doctor to court. A large number of expert witnesses then gave various points of view on his condition. These were divided, however, between those who thought he was malingering, those who believed he was suffering from neurasthenia, and those who thought it was a simple case of hysteria. Despite the doctor's admitting that he had applied electricity to this patient's face he was acquitted, the journal noting smugly that 'were this held to constitute legal cruelty, medical practitioners would be in frequent danger of being subjected to charges of this kind', noting also that he had been an unreliable witness.

Elsewhere, in official circles at least, suspicion sometimes conquered common sense. The author of Canada's official medical history of the war wrote: 'Under cover of these vague and mysterious symptoms the malingerer found refuge, and impressed a stigma upon those who were suffering from a real malady.'[73] As we shall see, two theatres of the war provided ample opportunity for a closer study of the problem; but even so, this still did little to weaken the official disdain for the shell-shocked as malingers by another name.

Endnotes

1 Hew Strahan, *The Outbreak of the First World War*, Oxford University Press, 2004, p. vi.
2 Raftery, *Marks of War*, p. 6.
3 E. Jones and S. Wessely, 'Psychiatric Battle Casualties: an Intra- and Interwar Comparison', *British Journal of Psychiatry*, vol. 178, 2001, p. 242. DAH was a term that was also used during the South African War. During the Gallipoli campaign 120 DAH cases were admitted to hospital.
4 For a discussion on reasons as to why this was the case, see Tyquin, *Gallipoli: the Medical War.*
5 Thomson, 'Status, Manpower and Mental Fitness', p. 151.
6 See Tyquin, *Gallipoli: the Medical War.*
7 Observations by Sir Harry Maudsley, Egypt 1916, pp. 2–3. AWM 27 376/3.
8 Thomson, 'Status, Manpower and Mental Fitness', p. 154.
9 Letter to the Deputy Repatriation Commissioner, 5 January 1937. SP 948/1 G530, NAA (Sydney).
10 See Appendix One.
11 W.G. MacPherson, (ed.), *History of the Great War Based on Official Documents: Diseases of the War*, vol. II, p. 2. However on page three in the same history there is this summary of 'mental' cases: '1,884 hospital admissions (officers and other ranks) from Gallipoli 1915—British Troops only). Totals are for: "neurasthenia, shell shock, hysteria etc", "epilepsy", vertigo, headache etc, "other diseases of the nervous system" and "mental diseases". Deaths:11; invalided from service:125; discharged to duty: 1,748.
12 McPherson, *History of the Great War*, vol. II, p. 3.
13 Butler, *Official History*, vol. III, p. 79.
14 McPherson, *History of the Great War*, vol. II, p. 4.
15 Butler, *Official History*, vol. III, pp. 101–2.
16 'Report on Observations of Invalid Boards by Colonel Sir Harry Maudsley', September 1918, p. 14. AWM 27 376/24.
17 Butler, *Official History*, vol. III, table 56, p. 939.
18 Letter from C.K. Parkinson MC (formerly a Lieutenant-Colonel in the AAMC, Senior Medical Boarding Officer) to A.G. Butler, 5 November 1935. He was then the Senior Medical Officer (NSW) for the Repatriation Department. AWM 41 [54].
19 Stone, 'Shellshock and the Psychiatrists', p. 249.
20 W. Beattie-Smith, 'Address in Neurology and Psychiatry', Ninth Session, Australasian Medical Congress, Sydney, 1911, *Australasian Medical Gazette*, 20 October 1911, p. 562.
21 Garton, *The Cost of War: Australians Return*, p. 156.
22 Feudtner, 'Minds the Dead Have Ravished...', p. 410.
23 Originally titled: 'Shell Shock and War Neuroses in the War of 1914–1918', Butler changed the relevant chapter title in his history to 'Moral and Mental Disorders in the War of 1914–1918'.
24 Raftery *Marks of War*, p. 16.
25 Extract from Major J. T. Jones (RMO 47th Battalion) Narrative, n.d. re Pozières August 1916. AWM 41/658.
26 Stone, 'Shellshock and the Psychiatrists', p. 251.
27 Cited in Butler, *Official History*, vol. III, p. 83.
28 R. Prior and T. Wilson, *The Somme*, University of New South Wales Press, 2005, p. 244.
29 Lance-Corporal A.A. Barwick. Diary entry for 26 April 1916. MSS 1493. Mitchell Library, Sydney (hereafter ML).
30 The sample admittedly is a small one and consists of infantry privates, but it represents a larger random sample of forty or so case files.
31 File: 14/8956. State Records of New South Wales.
32 File: 14/8956. State Records of New South Wales.
33 File: 14/8957. Case Papers (Australian Military Forces) 1915–1920. State Records of New South Wales.

34 File: 14/8956. State Records of New South Wales.
35 File: 14/8957. Case Papers (Australian Military Forces) 1915–1920. State Records of New South Wales.
36 MacPhail, *Official History of the Canadian Forces in the Great War 1914–1919: the Medical Services*, p. 276.
37 H. Binneveld, *From Shell Shock to Combat Stress: A Comparative History of Military Psychiatry*, Amsterdam University Press, 1997, p. 86.
38 Butler, *Official History*, vol. III, p. 107.
39 C. E. W Bean, Diary 116, Among the troops of 58th Battalion, Thursday evening 8 August 1918. AWM 3DRL 606.
40 H. Wiltshire, 'A Contribution to the Etiology of Shell Shock', *The Lancet*, vol. II, 17 June 1916, pp. 1207–12.
41 *Medical Annual*, Wright, Bristol, 1917, p. 461.
42 Butler, *Official History*, vol. III, pp. 118–19.
43 Deane, *Shook Over Hell*, p. 30.
44 SECRET Letter to DMS 4th Army from Lieutenant-Colonel H B. Sawer for Surgeon-General Slogett (RAMC), HQ 4th Army, 17 November 1916. AWM 41 649.
45 J. W. Springthorpe, 'Twelve Months' Service at the Front', *MJA*, 29 April 1916, p. 6.
46 A.G. Butler, 'The Treatment of "The Effort Syndrome"', *MJA*, 31 May 1941, p. 668.
47 J. Bostock, and E. Jones, *The Nervous Soldier: A Handbook for the Prevention, Detection and Treatment of Nervous Inability in War*, Queensland University Press, Brisbane, 1943, p. 32.
48 Butler, *Official History*, vol. III, p. 463.
49 Thomas Lewis, *The Soldier's heart and the Effort Syndrome*, 2nd edn, Shaw & Sons, London, 1940, p. 6.
50 Butler, *Official History*, vol. III, p. 91.
51 W. James, *The Australian Army Medical Corps in Egypt*, H.K. Lewis, London, 1918, p. 97.
52 Binneveld, *From Shell Shock to Combat Stress*, p. 87.
53 File: 14/8958. State Records of New South Wales.
54 File: 14/8958. State Records of New South Wales.
55 MacPherson (ed.), *History of the Great War Based on Official Documents: Diseases of the War*, vol. II, p. 40.
56 Ibid.
57 In World War I the British Army executed 346 soldiers for various offences. It is believed that a number of these were for cowardice, but these men should probably have been treated as neurotic. T. Bogacz, 'War Neurosis and Cultural Change in England 1914–1922: the Work of the War Office Committee of Enquiry into "Shell-Shock"', *Journal of Contemporary History*, 24, 1989, p. 51*n*.
58 See Bean's *Official History of the Great War*, volumes III (pp. 940–1), V (pp. 27–33), and VI (pp. 486–7).
59 Leed, *No Man's Land*, p. 169.
60 Roger Cooter, 'Malingering in Modernity: Psychological Scripts and Adversarial Encounters during the First World War' in R. Cooter, M. Harrison and S. Sturdy (eds.), *War, Medicine and Modernity*, Stroud, 1999, p. 130.
61 Memorandum of 27 July 1915 from Brigadier-General Sinclair-MacLagan to Officer Commanding 10th Battalion. AWM 41 [649]. The punishment at the time for 'self mutilation' was two years' hard labour.
62 Case Papers (Australian Military Forces) 1915–1920, File 14/8957. State Records of New South Wales.
63 File: 14/8956. State Records of New South Wales.
64 File: 14.8656. State Records of New South Wales.
65 Butler, *Official History*, vol. III, table 26, p. 896. The real number is likely to be higher. No such incidents are officially listed for Dardanelles, Egypt, Mesopotamia or Palestine.

66 C. Corns and J. Hughes-Wilson, *Blindfold and Alone: British Military Executions in the Great War*, London, 2001, p. 309.
67 AWM 41 [588].
68 McPhail, *Official History of the Canadian Forces in the Great War 1914–1919: the Medical Services*, pp. 277–8.
69 R.J. Ramsay (ed.), *Hell, Hope and Heroes: Life in the Field Ambulance in World War 1*, Rosenberg, Dural, 2005, p. 85.
70 A. A. Barwick, diary entry 24 July 1916. ML MSS 1493.
71 Editorial: 'The Wastage from Incompleteness', *MJA*, 22 July 1916, p. 59.
72 Joanna Bourke, 'Shell Shock and Australian Soldiers in the Great War', *Sabretache*, vol. XXXVI, no. 3, July–September 1995, p. 3.
73 MacPhail, *Official History of the Canadian Forces in the Great War 1914–1919: the Medical Services*, p. 277.

Chapter Four
The World and the Individual's Place in it

Typically, shell shock is closely, if not indelibly, linked with the Western Front between 1915 and 1918. But Australian, British and other troops also suffered in that sideshow known as the 'Gallipoli campaign'. We look first into that theatre from the Australian perspective, before moving on to the larger picture in France and Belgium. Individual experiences highlight the private hell for those soldiers who found this static kind of warfare too much to deal with.

Gallipoli and Egypt 1915

Gallipoli is regarded as a coming of age for Australia. Together with other British dominions allies, the Australian Government acquiesced in sending thousands to their deaths on the grim shores of the Turkish peninsula. Generally, these soldiers (who were not yet called 'diggers') made a great impression with their dash and tenacity but, as the inertia of the landing stagnated into months of stalemate and the weather deteriorated, enthusiasm dwindled. For others, the very thought of action was too much for them. This sideshow to the Great War shared the two features that are often exclusively associated with the Western Front, but are almost never aired in discussions of the AIF in 1915: shell shock and malingering.

The deadlocked nature of this campaign is perhaps one of the keys to understanding the incidence of shell shock at Gallipoli. The imagery and the reality of the lack of manoeuvre and inertia that became a feature of the Western Front cannot be underestimated in this theatre of war either. 'For all ranks the very nature of battle on the Western Front, a static struggle dominated by machines where the individual counted for little, contributed greatly to widespread mental illness after November 1914 when the stalemate began.'[1] It did not take long for the connection to be made. 'It was generally recognised that neurosis was germane to trench warfare and the peculiar emotional states that were generated by stable siege war. It was precisely the immobilisation of combat that seemed to be the most basic underlying reality of the neurotic symptom.'[2] There were very few recorded cases of mental illness among Australian Light Horsemen during the Palestine campaign, one characterised by almost constant movement over vast distances, mobile operations that their immobile comrades in the trenches could only dream about. The experiences of Gallipoli and the Western Front—both campaigns notable for their lack of manoeuvre—underscore the connection between shell shock and fixed battlefields in which massed artillery could be brought to bear.

Neurosis and mental breakdown were not, of course, the preserve of the private soldier. One of the earliest cases to be recorded at Gallipoli occurred on the day of the landing at Anzac Cove in April 1915. This incident concerned a senior officer, one Lieutenant-Colonel W.G. Patterson. His behaviour on the beach was so bizarre that Colonel John Gellibrand and Colonel Smith, the Assistant Provost Marshal, had to take him aside and place a guard on him. Patterson 'was hunting around with a revolver in his hand looking for General Bridges [the Australian commander] to kill him.'[3] He had acted strangely on the transport ship by walking up and down 'with a revolver in hand ordering some bakery fellows to disembark with their equipment.' The good colonel, a Boer War veteran, was consequently boarded with the diagnosis 'nervous instability'. Official proceedings stated that, at Anzac Cove on 25 April, he 'suffered from neurasthenia "unconscious for two days"' and he appeared to prove this diagnosis by dying 'on 19 May 1916 from "neurasthenia."'[4] The actions of other Australian junior commanders had less justification.

Officers did not have to resort to the self-inflicted wound to escape the front. At a time when every available man was needed, the contempt for the few who fled is evident in a diary entry by the commander of the 4th Australian Field Ambulance, L. J. Beeston. 'The number of officers clearing out is not commendable. One cannot wonder at the men squibbing it, one is more and more surprised at officers in whom we would have placed every confidence before the war and they are so bare-faced about it.'[5] As the strain of trench warfare and the toll from the ever-vigilant Turkish snipers grew, more soldiers did their best to escape Gallipoli. 'During the night nine self-inflicted wounded men were transferred to me from the 6th Field Ambulance.'[6] Even reinforcements were prone to breakdown. Sergeant H. Woods of the 4th Australian Field Ambulance noted in his diary: 'A newly arrived man (16th Battalion) purposely blew off his foot, and was detained in custody.'[7]

A New Zealand RMO at Gallipoli described a patient at the other end of the spectrum. The man was young and fought in the trenches, and is now recognisable as a typical picture of war neurosis, a term unknown on Anzac. Private K was 18 and considered undersized. He participated in an attack on a strategic position (Hill 60) and went forward with his platoon commander and ten men. They took cover under a hedge and began to fire. Private K found that he could not discharge his rifle or even put it to his shoulder. He was then told by his officer to crawl back to the forward trench, which he did. That evening his pulse was recorded as 120, his temperature 100 degrees. He could not walk in a straight line and his whole body trembled and twitched uncontrollably. His hands were tightly clenched together and when the doctor made him loosen them, the soldier's hands shook violently. He could not sleep and every shot made him jump or twitch. He admitted that he could never face fire again. The medical officer wrote that 'this boy may be called a coward, but it is to be noted that he advanced under heavy machinegun fire and did not retire until ordered. I believe his nervous system, like his body, *weak in the first place* [emphasis added], has been permanently shattered.'[8]

A nursing sister also related a bedside experience of another young shell-shocked patient evacuated from Anzac. May Tilton remembered nursing a 20-year-old 'who regained his reason but lost his voice [known as aphonia]. He told me in the faintest whisper that he saw his two elder brothers killed one day on the Peninsula. He went mad and wanted to rush the Turks' trenches; remembered being prevented; then knew no more. He could not understand why he could not talk.'[9]

'Disordered Action of the Heart' (DAH), as previously mentioned, was a vague syndrome which was little understood despite its being part of military medical lore in Britain for decades prior to the First World War. According to the Australian medical historian, A. G. Butler, during the nine months of the Gallipoli campaign 287 cases were diagnosed 'DAH' and 'evacuated from Gallipoli, a rate of 13.2 per cent per thousand per annum.' Butler researched and wrote his volumes of medical history over a period of fifteen years from the early 1930s. As late as 1943 he remained reluctant to attribute DAH to a psychological cause. He wrote that '...it seems difficult to escape the conclusion that the physical factors on Gallipoli, or at least the environment, were as much a "cause" of DAH there as the neurotic predisposition postulated today by psychiatrists.'[10] By early 1915 the Australians had established their major base hospitals in Egypt and No. 2 Australian General Hospital (AGH) in Cairo received most psychiatric casualties from Gallipoli. One of the doctors there, Major Archie Campbell, noted that: '...attacks of definite insanity were little if at all more frequent among our troops than they would be in a similar body of men under peace conditions.'[11] This was also the experience of many doctors in France. Between February and September 1915, No.2 AGH admitted eighty-one men classified as 'nervous'. In keeping

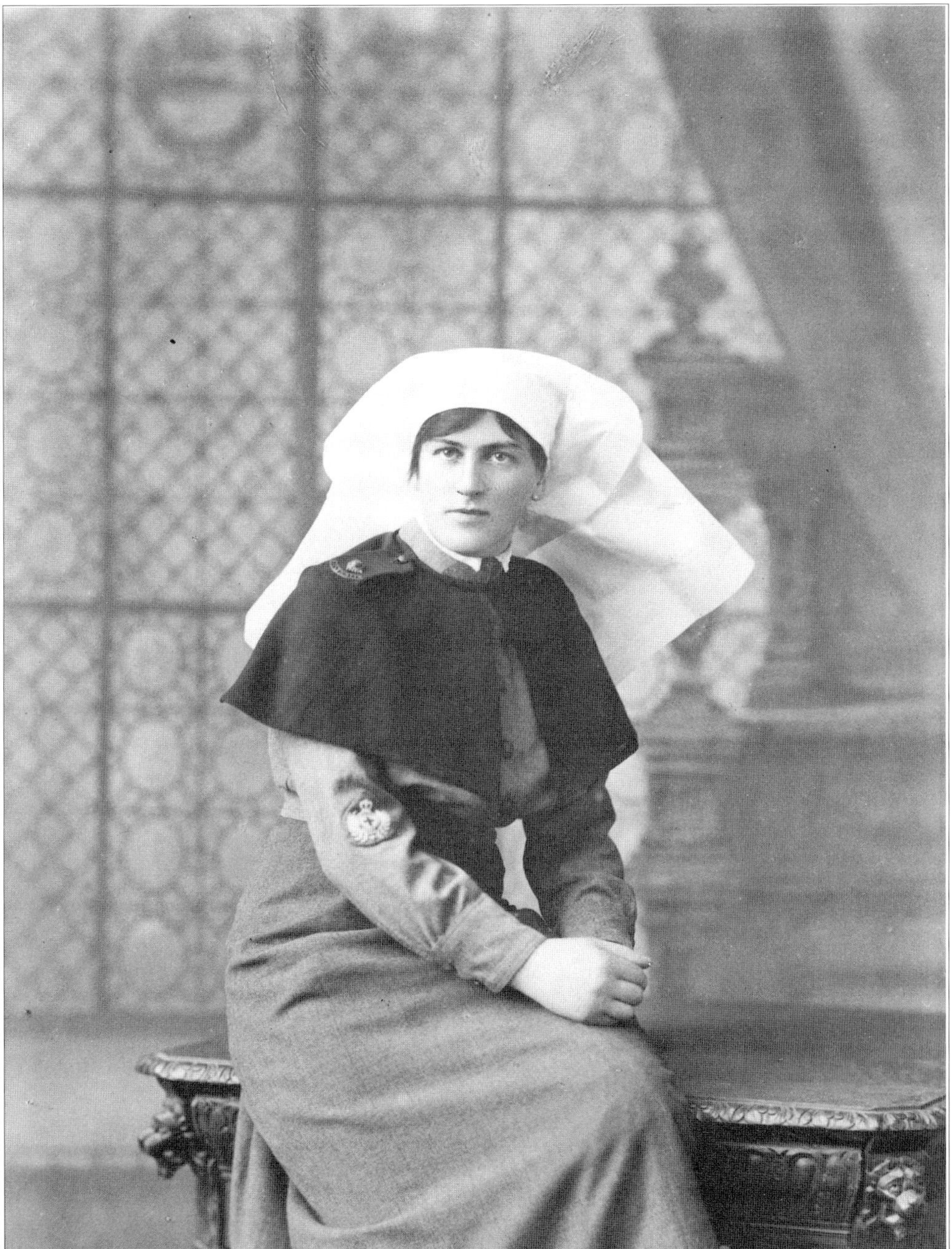

A striking portrait of Staff Nurse Frances MacKellar of the AANS, c.1917. She was one of several staff who cared for mental patients at the No. 3 Australian Auxiliary Hospital at Dartford, England. (AWM PO4115.001)

with the vague diagnostic labels of the time, it was not uncommon for men admitted with sunstroke to be classified as suffering neurasthenia.

One medical officer in Cairo remembered 'a number of youths and men whose mental capacity was so far below the average that they could not be trained into efficient soldiers. A few of these cases of partial dementia in youths had developed during active service in Egypt or at Anzac, but in the majority of cases from the general aspect of the patient and his history it was evident that he always had been half-witted and unable to earn his living in civil life. One or two examples of actual insanity (recurrent mania and melancholia) came before me and there was the history in these cases of a previous attack in an asylum.'[12] Another AAMC officer working in Egypt in 1915 was also of the opinion that malingering should never be far from the doctor's mind when making a diagnosis. 'There is, however, a type of case much more difficult to handle than the malingerer—the man with a tendency to neurasthenia or hysteria, who exaggerates his symptoms, and who is subconsciously endeavouring to prove that he is really worse than the medical officer thinks he is.'[13] He admitted, however, that it was often difficult to discern malingerers and 'the element of nervous disposition.'

In 1916 Major A.W. Campbell recorded his observations in a paper which was published in the *Medical Journal of Australia*. He categorised psychological casualties into four types: first, there were neuroses 'involving the motor apparatus and common sensibility'; then neuroses involving 'the special senses and the faculty of speech'; third was 'neurasthenia' and other conditions; and finally, minor psychoses, 'mental stupor' and 'insanity'. Significantly, he added what was to become the classic medical opinion throughout the war: 'Time after time, on going into the family and personal histories of such cases, we found evidence of neuropathic or psychopathic infirmity, and this was the fundamental cause of their *downfall* [emphasis added].'[14] This view was strongly held, especially by medical officers, at a time when the eugenics movement was gaining popularity in Europe and throughout the British Empire. While it is true, as has been stated, that a number of soldiers did indeed have a questionable mental history, they did not, as was often suggested in the professional literature, make up the majority of shell shock casualties.

The following extract is worth quoting at length not only for the light it sheds on the psychological aspect of the Gallipoli campaign, but also as a means of highlighting the fragility of surviving statistics. It comes from one of A.G. Butler's unpublished drafts for his official medical history of the war:

> The uncertainty in the classification, however, especially at that stage of the war [1915], and the changes afterwards introduced into it, make exact comparisons impossible. The diagnosis 'shell shock' seems to have been used during the Gallipoli Campaign as well as 'shock' and 'traumatic neurasthenia.' But the term 'NYDN' [Not Yet Diagnosed-Nervous] which after 1916 was employed on the Western Front for every case of 'nervous breakdown' in which the exciting cause might not have been shell shock was not in use on Gallipoli. The result is that, though the student would expect to find in Gallipoli heavier wastage from the disorder classed as 'neurasthenia' (as the result of long continued 'conflict') and on the Western Front a larger proportion from other forms of 'nervous breakdown' that derive from more definitely positive and violent emotional traumatic—through shell burst, burial under debris, and so forth—this cannot be proved from the figures.[15]

We come now to the geographic apotheosis of shell shock in popular memory: the Western Front.

The Western Front

In his discussion of the Western Front, one scholar has suggested that 'soldiers became demoralised and "quite incapable of any excitement" once they recognized that "individuality in the struggle was lost." The modern soldier was pitted against anonymous agents and his aggression was also incognito.'[16] This is a theme echoed by many other historians, writers and even artists. However there is little documentary evidence to suggest mental depression on any large scale in the AIF after the massive withdrawal from the Gallipoli peninsula in December 1915. There was little excitement but no loss of individuality even though the Turks had been at times a very visible and hardly anonymous enemy. There was certainly disappointment that they had to leave many of their mates behind for no gain. The withdrawal came at a period during the wider war in which, apart from naval gunfire, little technology was deployed, unlike the artillery Armageddon that would evolve in France and Belgium from 1916.

A senior AAMC officer wrote of the newly formed Anzac Corps' first blooding in the Somme during July and August 1916 and of its initial shell shock cases: 'The fighting which took place on the battlefield of Pozieres was of that severe, sustained nature calculated to bring out any tendencies to nervous strain or breakdown from shock. As every trench carried by our men was not only gained in the face of the fiercest fire from machine guns and H.E. [high explosive] shrapnel, and when gained was held for days and nights always subjected to an incessant tornado of H.E. fire from heavy guns.'[17] However, Butler, in reading RMOs' reports from heavy engagements like the Pozières battle, thought that he could disprove any psychic link with the resultant mental casualties. He confidently concluded that '"shell shock" as a "wound", in the physical sense...is a figment', and suggested a substitute term 'battle shock.'[18] In that same winter however, and not far away, the New Zealanders were also suffering from the unremitting pressures of this war and 'their diaries chart a growing irritability until the inevitable breakdown.'[19]

There were several problems in dealing appropriately with war neuroses in the field: firstly their causation was still poorly understood; secondly, most RMOs had no training in what then passed for psychology; and third, in the rush of casualties and amid the fog of war, there was not the time required to properly assess and treat these men;[20] fourth, there was the need to isolate many such cases to prevent panic; and lastly, as previously mentioned, there was increasing pressure on doctors as military officers to be firm with soldiers they viewed as treading the fine line between shell shock and malingering. The RMO was seen as healer, policeman and judge. 'The war helped render a problem of discipline (bounded by law and morality) into one of psychiatry (bounded by medicine).'[21] The vast majority of medical officers, who had until the war been citizen practitioners used to the comfortable limits set by the Hippocratic Oath, would have found their first front-line experiences unsettling. 'When presented with a soldier evacuated with shell shock, the doctors in uniform suddenly found themselves mediating between these two radically different concepts of individual responsibility [i.e. to the soldier-patient or to the army-employer]. In many ways, the conflict over responsibility was the central issue of managing shell shock.'[22]

No-one was immune from the appalling conditions of the Western Front. Lieutenant-Colonel J.W. Springthorpe, in poetic mood, described the destruction in his unpublished memoirs of the war. In describing the AIF fighting around Pozières the manuscript says: 'There for the first time shell shock falls like an avalanche on thousands.'[23] And so it was to be, in varying degrees and in different parts of the line, for the rest of the war. Here are some typical case studies:

Private S, a 31-year-old photographer, was blown up by a shell at Pozières and sent to the United Kingdom. Several months later he was reported to be 'Very nervous and hysterical cannot speak about the accident without crying. Is not likely to be fit for some time.'[24]

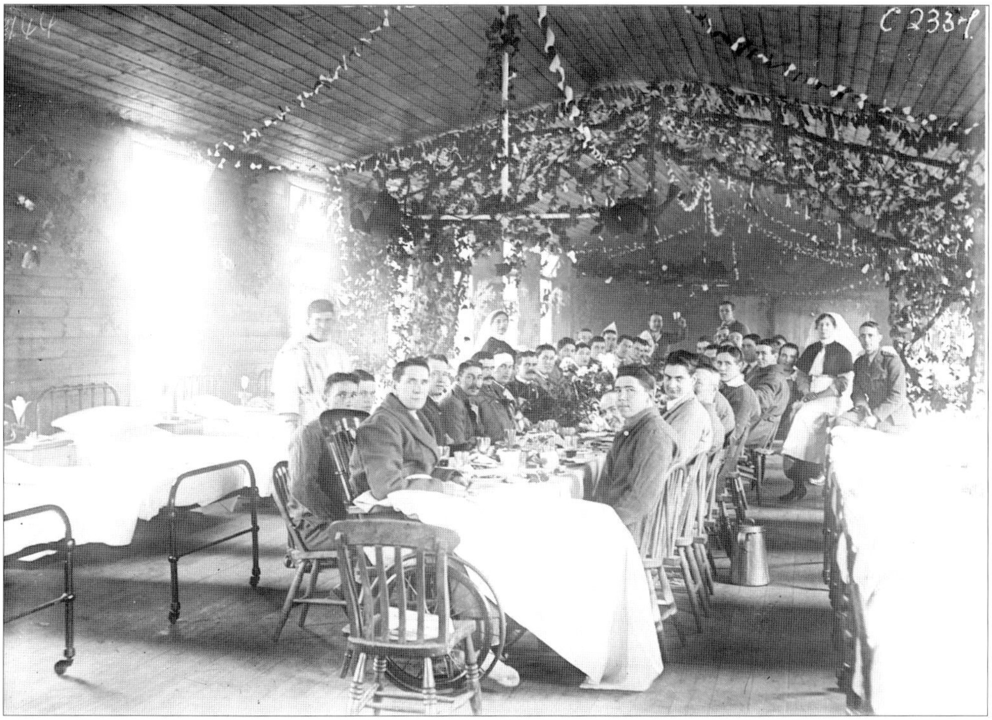

Patients of a shell shock ward at No. 3 Australian Auxiliary Hospital, Dartford, Christmas 1916. Military medicine was still struggling for answers at this period of the war. (AWM C02337)

Private C of the 54th Battalion, a former electrician aged 31, had enlisted in June 1914 and served in Egypt and on the Western Front. In France in 1917 he was treated for shell shock following an incident which left him unconscious for 24 hours. By late January 1918 he was still a patient at Dartford, with 'neurological symptoms and stammering.'[25]

Private W from the 3rd Battalion, aged 47 years, had enlisted in January 1916. He was admitted for 'War Neurosis—shell shock' after being blown up at Bapaume on 10 April 1917 and remaining unconscious for four days. He was sent to various hospitals in the UK before being repatriated and taken to Broughton Hall in Sydney. 'Has not been able to walk since then. Continuous wheeze.'[26]

Gunner Butcher had enlisted in June 1915 and, while in France during 1916, he was blown up three times 'the third [not surprisingly] effected [sic] him badly.' He was evacuated to England and saw the inside of several hospitals before suffering a relapse. He complained of stabbing pains in the head, was 'easily excitable and perspires a good deal and is very shaky. He dreams sometimes about the battle hearing the explosions and noise etc and sometimes he feels as if the bed is pulled from him or is falling over a precipice.'[27]

Private A, a miner from the 17th Battalion, had enlisted in May 1915. He was blown up twice in three days. He was repatriated to Sydney in May 1918 and admitted to No. 4 AGH at Randwick. 'Suffered from insomnia, was shaky and upset easily by sudden noises.' He was moved to Broughton Hall Asylum in June that year 'still nervous, starts at sudden noises.'[28]

Private J of the 13th Battalion, aged 30, was in a trench when a shell exploded overhead, concussing him and rupturing an eardrum. He was diagnosed with 'Anxiety neurosis as a result of shock.' On admission to hospital this man 'was extremely depressed and miserable. He showed by every action, movement and facial expression extreme nervous tension. He talks absurd and gesticulates as if conversing to real beings.'[29]

The scale, the conditions, the sheer magnitude and mix of artillery and vehicles and supplies presented a new experience for the AIF which had arrived from the pocket handkerchief battlefield of Gallipoli where the enemy's heavy guns were so few that they had been given nicknames. On the Somme in September 1916 'Lt. Colonel E.A. Harris, disabled by shell-shock in no-man's land on 19 July had confessed to Brigadier General "Pompey" Elliott that after such an unnerving experience he doubted he could face another battle.'[30] Elliott, a much-loved senior Australian commander, himself succumbed to suicide long after the war was over, although the exact cause is open to speculation. On 17 November 1916, in the same area of the front, Bean 'noted in his diary "a chance remark" to the effect that "they say the Australian infantry are standing it very badly."' Bean admitted to being 'shocked with the look of the men'. For the first time he had 'passed an Australian Bn [battalion] without seeing a single smile on any man's face.' [31]

'It was the set piece battles, Verdun, the Somme, and in some more aggressive zones of routine combat, that casualties multiplied alarmingly, the result of violent surroundings, physical exhaustion, nervous and emotional strain.'[32] Years after the war, in a letter to Arthur Butler, a former medical officer made an interesting observation and put forward a rarely articulated hypothesis: 'It was remarked by the officers in my ambulance that we never saw a *wounded* soldier with shell shock. In other words his psychological difficulties had been solved by his wound, and by the time he had reached the Field Ambulance he considered that he was safe for the next few months.'[33] Unfortunately the lack of statistics makes probing this hypothesis difficult.

Australian troops were 'blooded' and traumatised particularly severely in the fighting around Pozières in July and August and on the Somme during 1916. According to the RMO of the 2nd Brigade, Captain H. R. J. Harris, who was one of the men in the thick of it at Pozières, there were many cases of 'shell shock'. In evacuating these mental casualties he did not consider it mattered much if the cause was one of 'stark fear or genuine "shell shock"'. He understood that the former had to be evacuated to the field ambulance because of 'the disastrous moral effect of a badly frightened man on his comrades.'[34] From Butler's perspective, these Pozières casualties during August could be classified into two categories. The first and smaller group 'were mentally and morally neuropathic' (by which he meant psychopathic) and 'whose psychic make-up pre-disposed or even pre-ordained them' to 'nervous breakdown'; and a second group of men who were sufficiently resilient to ensure that, with suitable treatment, 'they would recover from any save the most severe mental strains and shock.'[35] Once again the moral aspect assumes prominence in what would be seen nowadays as a strictly clinical assessment.

But while assessing the larger tactical picture, Butler proved perceptive in realising that aspects of the fighting on the Somme could provide him with a means of understanding the triggers behind these neuroses. There he identified three elements 'in the psychical environment' that for him stood out particularly. The first involved the physically traumatic aspect of the offensive weapons employed, especially high explosive shelling, while crucially, the second was 'the largely passive and impersonal nature of the battle experience'. The third element was what he described as the 'degeneration' of the offensive into 'a crude contest in attrition devoid of "surprise" or tactical refinement.' In this environment it became increasingly difficult for an individual soldier 'to regard his tasks as part of an intelligent plan.'[36] Butler had already coined the term 'battle shock' for the medical outcome of this lethal mix and was astute enough to identify the forced passivity and helplessness of otherwise robust individuals in what was becoming an artillery war on a massive scale as a contributing factor in mental breakdown.

There were differences in approaches and diagnoses among the allies. 'While both French and American Army medical services managed to develop a policy of positive expectancy towards traumatic neurosis, which assisted quick, full recovery, the British did not.'[37] Not unnaturally the British evacuated their first cases of 'combat fatigue' direct to England—just across the channel. In July 1916 Lieutenant-Colonel Charles Myers, consulting psychologist to the BEF 'persuaded the medical authorities to treat them at base hospitals in France.' Crucially, and this was to be the experience in the next war, 'the proximity to England and the expectation of evacuation home tended to reinforce symptoms. Thus with Myers (who later fell out with the military hierarchy) as a key instigator, there began a more effective regime of keeping troops at or near the front and treating them at special forward medical centres. Generally the results were significantly better.'[38]

The proximity to the fighting generally kept these 'casualties' near their own units, and therefore still part of a fighting force. The authorities found that, by officially regarding shaken or exhausted troops as simply over-tired while otherwise perfectly healthy, these troops could be readily re-assimilated into front-line units after only a few days' rest. Long evacuations to the rear only reinforced symptoms of sickness and feelings of mental fragility for many. In 1918 J.W. Springthorpe, who had been in charge of war neurotics at No. 3 AGH since November 1916, acknowledged the French lead in front-line military psychology: 'The French whose definition was earlier and methods more thorough...combined our traumatic and shell-shock under the different heading of "*neuropsychiatric, emotionel, commotionel* [commotion equated with concussion]."[39] They treated the patients in separate hospitals and in a different manner and left the patients corresponding to our "neurasthenics" and "psychasthenics" to be dealt with either in general or other hospitals.'[40]

In terms of sophisticated medical treatment, particularly in rear areas, the AIF was largely dependent on the much larger, if still stretched, resources of the RAMC. Front-line 'treatment' of such men was largely haphazard. For troops who were simply over-tired and 'fed-up', the simple expedient of sending them to the rear of the line for a few days with good food, warm shelter and a bed was enough to see them return to the trenches without undue stress. However, for RMOs in forward areas, and even the doctors in field ambulances and other line medical elements in the rear who 'often lacked any specialist training; the most common definition of cure remained the cessation of visible symptoms.'[41] Typically for the victim these symptoms included some or all of these: uncontrollable tremors, stupor, temporary blindness or deafness, partial paralysis (usually of a hand or limb) and spontaneous crying. According to Colonel D. McWhae, it was not until early in 1919 that a wholly Australian psychotherapeutic department was established at Weymouth under an officer who had received 'a course of instruction' in suggestive treatment at the Seale Hayne Neurological Hospital.[42]

By 1918 and with the increasing tempo of the huge set-piece battles that now raged along the front, shell shock and other psychiatric casualties continued to worry senior Australian medical officers, even though many of these psychological casualties were, with the new treatment regime, only lost to units for short periods. 'Altogether in the first twenty days there were over two thousand cases of shell shock admitted, constituting nearly 20% of the total admissions for casualties from the battlefield.'[43] Most were returned from rest stations to their units within forty-eight hours. Writing towards the very end of the war, a medical officer admitted that the Australian RMOs and medical officers attached to various field ambulances went into the Somme offensive with a very ill defined, preconceived idea of shell shock. Once there and meeting 'the results of intense artillery concentration for the first time we all allowed men to pass through our stations, men whom undoubtedly we should retain under present conditions.'[44] Medicine and military were both wiser than they had been in 1915 and lessons had been assimilated with good effect—especially for the majority of front-line troops. We have had a brief glimpse of how the shell-shocked were dealt with, but the following accounts offer some different perspectives either from soldiers who dealt with neurotic mates or the men themselves.

Individual Experiences

There is usually no more revealing description of a shell-shocked casualty than the notes of the treating doctors. Rather than simply recording clinical observations, they often provide context for the soldier's own experiences. Here are a few that speak for themselves—some with particular poignancy—two from Gallipoli and five from the Western Front.

Private A of the 18th Battalion, a former fireman, had enlisted in June 1915 and later suffered shell shock at Pozières. Before this he had been buried on the Gallipoli peninsula and then three times in July and August in France during 1916. He was invalided in October 1916 from Ypres complaining of a distressing headache. He was described as 'Expression anxious, general tremor of head and limbs.'[45] Fred, a former hospital orderly, was another mature private soldier in the 4th Battalion who had enlisted early in 1915. He had embarked for Egypt and was at Gallipoli for eleven weeks when he was blown up by a bomb at Lone Pine and hurled against the side of a trench. Still unconscious, he was evacuated to Cairo where he remained for twelve months. In September 1916 he was deployed to the Somme and, along with several other men, he was 'blown up' at Bullecourt. He was dug out and remained unconscious for two hours before being evacuated to various hospitals in France and England and then repatriated to Australia in September 1917. On admission to the Military Asylum at Broughton Hall in Sydney he was 'still nervous and noises affect him, when excited gets tremulous and he feels uncertain gets flurried and nervous when crossing the streets. Has headaches.'[46] After 1917 he is lost to the sight of the historian.

Lance-Corporal B, a 26-year-old railway fireman, had fought all through the Gallipoli campaign before proceeding to France. In July 1916 he was wounded in the back and legs. Sent to hospital in France and then to England, he was away for about five months before returning to duty. Six months later he contracted some type of fever and was again admitted to hospital in France and then evacuated to England for four months before once again resuming duty. Eleven months later his 'nerves gave way' and he was sent back to hospital and returned to England where he was in hospital for some time before being 'boarded' to Australia.[47] Anyone trying to glimpse the state of this man's mind through this period of three years from such a peripatetic medical history can only speculate as to his mental health. Private G, a farmer, had enlisted in the 49th Battalion in 1915 and been returned to Australia in November 1917, aged 27. His medical record states that he had 'neurasthenia following shell shock and concussion.' He also began to suffer periodically from loss of memory and presented with mental confusion following a massive shell explosion in July 1916 at Albert on the Somme. After four to six months of 'normalcy' he developed fits and his clinical notes state that he was now 'excited and irresponsible in his actions while in England.'[48] Whatever treatment was meted out to him throughout the lengthy time-span between cause and 'cure' seems not to have had the desired effect. And yet 'G' was one of hundreds who shared this particular path.

Sapper H of the 7th Field Engineers was a 32-year-old carpenter who served in France. Repatriated to Australia in March 1917, he was admitted to Broughton Hall with shell shock. He could not remember anything prior to his admission to Dartford in England. 'H' had been part of a group of ten men blown up during an artillery barrage and had found himself the sole survivor. He told his doctor that 'all I know of France is what I dream.' He complained of headaches and spoke with a stammer. His body was so tremulous that he was forced to walk with a stick. His demons were 'very distressing dreams'.[49] Private C, 18 years old, a member of the 45th Battalion, had enlisted straight from school in 1915 and had been buried three times at Passchendaele, Bullecourt and Messines. His third brush with what was regarded as a horrid and feared way of dying proved the last straw and 'C' threatened to shoot two sergeants and attacked another non-commissioned officer at Bapaume. He was admitted to D Block at Netley Hospital in May 1918 bearing the label of 'delusional insanity' and was sent later to the Lord Derby Hospital. Not surprisingly, his clinical notes state that he 'does not sleep well at night because he dreams of events in France and the dreams worry him a lot...suffers from tremors.'[50] Such were the often physically unscarred human debris of this modern war.

As discussed earlier, C.E.W. Bean's role as recorder and narrator of Australia's experience in the Great War still holds a key place in shaping our collective memory. His 'invention' also continues to hold a peculiar sway over an Australian media increasingly prone to delivering misty-eyed expressions of nationalism. For all of this he was a consummate journalist and painstaking recorder of events for which the historian of this period must be grateful. He was often ideally placed to see at first hand the effect of high explosive shells, incessant heavy artillery fire and the other stressors of war on ordinary soldiers. Although there is little doubt that he was a sympathetic observer, he was in the business of shaping an exclusively Australian image for both domestic and foreign consumption.[51] This carefully crafted incarnation of nationhood had to be a tough and resilient one and, perhaps ironically, it is the warrior hero stereotype beloved of the First World War generation that Australia still celebrates. This is despite the obvious glossing-over of any hint of weakness, or failure, or doubt, and certainly madness.

It is not difficult to find examples of the way in which Bean used his raw material in his edited history of the war. The following is taken from a letter from Lieutenant J.A. Raws of the 23rd Battalion to his brother. Dated 12 August 1916, it describes a portion of the battle around Pozières in France. The italicised words are the only parts of the letter quoted by Bean in his published description:[52]

> The strain—you say it has not been too great for me—was really bad...Many other fine men broke to pieces. Everyone called it shell shock. But shell shock [concussion] is very rare. *What 90% get is justifiable funk [nerves, due to the collapse at the helm]—is* [sic] *self-control.* I felt fearful that my nerve was going at the very last morning...The OC went temporarily mad and deserted us...But the anxiety and horror of it I cannot tell you. I had to drive men who were in one trench ahead of us at one time, blocking the way, with my revolver.[53]

In an earlier (unpublished) letter from Raws to his sister and dated 8 August 1916, he had written:

> Our leader was shot before we arrived [in the trench] and the strain had sent two officers mad...We were being shot at all the time...I was buried twice, and thrown down several times—buried with dead and dying. The ground was covered with

> bodies in all stages of decay and mutilation and I would, after struggling free from the earth, pick up a body by me to lift him out with me and find him a decayed corpse. I pulled a head off—was covered in blood. The horror was indescribable...I've told you hardly anything.[54]

Bean, of course, could not publish such stuff, but it is a graphic depiction of the environment that contributed to soldiers' losing their mind—even if momentarily. The following paragraphs include a few more unpublished accounts taken from Bean's many personal notebooks. They provide an interesting contrast to the paucity of references subsequently made in his defining 'historical' rendering of events from 1915 to 1918.[55]

While himself at the front, Bean mentions two men who became shell shocked after an aeroplane dropped five bombs. Diary 179, dated 27 July 1917 and written at Trois Arbres: 'Started digging trench from Kirk's Strong Post. Still uncertain as to what was to be done—the suspense is very trying and men getting very nervy.' Diary 131, 17th Battalion at Pozières, 1 August 1916: 'The 19th Bn does not really know yet what happened. The men seem to have been upset by something; they turned or got into shell holes. The best officers or NCOs were at once hit trying to get them on.' Diary 130, 19th Battalion at Pozières, May 1916: 'Donolly went out through one of the sally ports and met them [stretcher party] bringing in Colonel Harris, blown up by a shell and suffering from shell shock.' 'Lt Orpen came in suffering from shell-shock—so only one officer left—Lt Cadden.' Then, in Diary 123, when Bean was probably in a better position to appreciate the effects of artillery at the front, he wrote of the 58th Battalion at Fromelles, 19–20 July 1916. In Diary 136 he described Pozières: 'The genuine shell shocks were a feature of Pozieres—each gun that went off affecting the men.' He then described the first Passchendaele battle in October 1916: Lt J. Monfries of the 34th Battalion suffering 'shell shock led pln during attack, knocked silly by shell [12/10/17]' (Diary 178). In the 44th Battalion 'Lt. O' Carroll on coming out to Hill 40 first time was badly shell shocked and has been in bed ever since' (Diary 175). Diary 141 noted on 20 October 1917 that the 50th Battalion's losses at Pozieres on 13 August 1916 amounted to '8 officers and 406 men, besides some shell shock.' Finally there is a little portrait of an individual casualty from the 8th Battalion at Pozières:

> At 5 am the [German] bombardment opened and continued all day increasing as the day went on till about 3 pm the word was sent back that the Germans were attacking from both flanks left and right...[Private] Traill was shooting at them for some time before being hit by a 5.9 [lb shell]. He was put in a cellar—and the

cellar was broken in [sic] by a shell—when he came to he was covered with bits of cellar. Then he was blown up on the stretcher.' (Diary 26)

Apparently this soldier survived his ordeal—at least psychologically.

But what of the soldiers for whom the war was not just a struggle for survival, but a day-to-day chore of appalling dimensions? Corporal George Faulkner was one of these men. A stretcher bearer with the 15th Australian Field Ambulance, he made numerous references to shell shock while his unit was deployed in France in 1916. Here are some, the first beginning while he was working in an Advanced Dressing Station on 16 July 1916:

> Had two cases of shock in particular who were painful to watch, just a bundle of nerves and ready to cow at the slightest noise.
>
> 20 July 1916 at the 32nd Aid Post:
>
> ...things were some [sic] hot—Fritz was dropping them [artillery shells] hard and swift all around, it was just raining shrapnel. The Regimental SBSs [stretcher bearers], who without a doubt are as brave as any man in the army, were either shot, fagged out or gone in the nerves.
>
> I consider no man could do justice to ghastly sights behind the parapet yesterday—the chaos—the dead in different attitudes, the wounded who are only distinguished by their moaning—the nerve broken soldier trying to do his duty at his post with dead all around them. It will be a nightmare to me at all times.
>
> 22 October 1916 near Albert:
>
> As we are lined up against rows of guns of every calibre, it is that deafening and nerve racking [sic] that I couldn't sleep.
>
> 27 October 1916, Bapaume:
>
> About a dozen of our [stretcher] bearers are put of action through Blighty's sprained ankles, shell shock etc. Three fellows that used to carry with me have gone off with shell shock...in my wildest dreams I never thought war meant anything like this.[56]

Nightmarish scenes like these have now entered the common experience of that war. It could be a shattering ordeal for any human mind. Joy Damousi wrote that Australians joined the war with fervour. Brought up like their British and European colleagues on 'a fare of nineteenth century stories that portrayed war as romantic, glamorous and heroic, young Australian men had no conception of battle, let alone of what trench warfare, shellfire or slaughter would be like.'[57] Disillusionment followed quickly.

The following are extracts from notes taken on the Somme during late 1916 and 1917 by Lance-Corporal A. J. Moore, also a stretcher bearer, but attached to the 8th Australian Field Ambulance. They illustrate the profundity of such disillusionment with this new, barbaric, unremitting type of battle:

> 23 October 1916, near Albert:
>
> Things are mighty rough for us, but how the poor devils of infantrymen stick it is beyond me. There are about 20 of our men sick and suffering from shell shock. It is an awful strain on all of us.
>
> 28 October 1916:
>
> A big number of bearers are sick or suffering from shell shock, so we had to fall back on the Nursing Section to give us a hand.
>
> 13 April 1917, near Bellevue farm:
>
> Fritz is shelling heavily...Just as they [a stretcher party] moved off a shell burst almost on top of them and I had to take Maggs' place as he got a bad dose of shell shock.[58]

The 'bad dose' referred to was probably of the concussive type as the writer, mimicking his seniors, seems to have used the meaning of shell shock freely—as both a physical and psychological problem.

Private Longord Colley-Priest, another stretcher bearer with the 8th Australian Field Ambulance, diarised his first experiences on the Western Front at Fromelles in July 1916: 'A chap has just been brought in and is sitting by my side, poor devil, his whole body is shaking, one would think he was shivering from the cold. His nerves must be shattered.'[59] In the following year Sergeant W. C. Watson of the 31st Battalion pondered over some of the other issues that seemed to be closely associated with the issue of shell shock: 'Reviewing little incidents, I cannot get it right how some NCOs have the nerve to take charge of men, knowing that they had not the courage of most of their men. I have seen some desert their section paralysed with nervousness or fear... During the day several men were effected [sic] by shell shock caused by shells bursting near them. It was pitiful to see the nervous wrecks of men being led out by the hand crouching in terror at the sound of any passing shell whether ours or the enemy's.'[60] Watson himself had also been present at several trench cave-ins and had a fear of being buried alive.

But one of the most reflective personal narratives concerning war neuroses is this one by Sapper Ernest De Mouncy. His calmness in a crisis may indicate what some might regard nowadays as symptomatic of post combat stress syndrome, a comparison we will return to.

> I went through a bad time in France. You cannot without being there realise the awfulness of it all & I can hardly realise it yet that I am really homeward bound. How on earth anyone gets out of it I cannot understand. It is one continuous roar of guns and big ones at that. At first you take no notice of them bursting overhead & all round, but after a time, when you have seen fellows falling all about & you get blown up once or twice then you become to get a bit windy.

During his voyage home to Australia, a destroyer escort dropped some depth charges, the impact of which was felt in De Mouncy's troop-ship. Panic ensued, as the soldiers on board thought the ship had been torpedoed. 'There was a stampede for the boat. By the time I had got out of my hammock there was not a soul left below but myself...Strange to say I did not experience the slightest feeling of fear and was taking things calmly.' De Mouncy had been badly gassed at Villers-Bretonneux and evacuated on 1 June 1918.[61]

Those whose private demons could not be exorcised by medical science were placed on ships specially staffed and fitted out for the long journey back to Australia. Such voyages were not without their own distractions, as occurred on the journeys described in the following accounts:

> The officer [Captain W.E. Julien, a chaplain] was given a cabin to himself. He was suffering from delusions and disappeared from HMT *Miltiades* in May 1917 while returning to Australia. He got off at Sierra Leone, was captured three weeks later and sent to Cape Town on 16 June...and admitted to Wynberg Hospital 4 July 1917. He escaped from there on 9 July 1917 but was again captured after wandering over 400 miles and was placed on board the HMT *Euripides* on 26 August 1917.
>
> On the night of 7 August 1917 while in Port at Sierra Leone 114 Pte M. Clenaghan 26 Btn attempted suicide by hanging, he was prevented by [a medical sergeant] who was on night duty. Second attempt 5 September 1917, prevented by [another medical attendant]. This patient and several others have been under special individual observation throughout the voyage.[62]

On the same voyage, of the fifty-eight patients aboard, five were suffering from shell shock, and two of these had been buried alive in mine explosions. 'Four of them have recovered mentally and physically, and one still remains delusional though physically well.'[63]

What is revealed behind the tough, devil-may-care AIF of legend is that there was in its ranks another type of man who, while he could rise to the occasion, was less robust than the mass of battle-hardened soldiers around him. As we have seen there is also ample evidence to suggest that even the toughest men had a limit to their mental and physical endurance, and it seemed that the youngest were most vulnerable to psychological shocks. This comment, again from an experienced senior AAMC officer, was prescient despite the evident condescension: 'The younger men at the front were a failure. I satisfied myself that men of 19 and 20 cannot stand physical or mental strain such as they are called upon to stand. I saw some boys not much over 17, and it is doubtful if they will ever be the same again, owing to the shock and stress.'[64] Ten years later it was this age group that would emerge, belatedly perhaps, suffering from the mental scars of their experiences. This is not to say, however, that little was done to help them during the war itself as we shall see.

Endnotes

1 Bogacz, 'War Neurosis and Cultural Change in England 1914–1922, p. 33. This is a point also made in the most recent assessment of the battles in the Somme during 1916. The authors suggest that military historians are still 'devoted to the notion that the outcome of even the largest conflicts is determined by the skill and heroism of the rank and file infantry', but it was actually 'the mass produced, long-range killing machines that now dominated the battlefield.' Prior and Wilson, *The Somme*, p. 117.

2 Leed, *No Man's Land*, p. 181.

3 Bridges was later killed by a Turkish sniper.

4 Letter of 4 May 1931 from A.G. Butler to Major A.J. Withers, compiler of Medical History. AWM 41 [279]. In the official Australian war history (vol. I, p.77) C.E.W. Bean tactfully noted that 'Patterson broke down under the trials and worry of the Landing...'

5 Quoted in Tyquin, *Gallipoli: The Medical War*, p. 38. See also pp. 146–9.

6 War Diary entry, 5th Field Ambulance, 11 December 1915. AWM 41 26/48.

7 Diary entry 10 November 1915, Sergeant (later Lieutenant) H.H.V. Woods, 4th Field Ambulance. AWM 3DRL 358.

8 'August 1915, RMO's Report' in A.D. Carberry, *The New Zealand Medical Service in the Great War 1914–1918*, Whitecombe & Tombs, Wellington, 1924, pp. 109–110.

9 May Tilton, *The Grey Battalion*, Angus & Robertson, Sydney, 1934, p. 15.

10 Butler, *Official History*, vol. III, p. 86.

11 Ibid., p. 87.

12 Observations by Sir H. Maudsley, Egypt 1916, p. 2. AWM 27 376/3.

13 J.W. Barrett, *A Vision of the Possible*, H. K. Lewis, London, 1919, p. 108.

14 A.W. Campbell, 'Remarks on some Neuroses and Psychoses in War', *MJA*, 15 April 1916, pp. 319 and 323.

15 A. G. Butler, 'Medical History Drafts', vol. III, Chapter 2, p. 49. AWM 44 16/4 Part I.

16 J. Bourke, *An Intimate History of Killing: Face-to-Face Combat in Twentieth Century Warfare*, Grantor Books, London, 1999, p. 249.

17 Summary by Colonel C.C. Manifold, DDMS Australian Corps, to A.G. Butler, 1 February 1918, p. 1. AWM 41 [659].

18 Butler, *Official History*, vol. III, p. 104.

19 Pugsley, *The Face of Hell*, p. 171.

20 As the British official medical history makes clear: '...under the conditions existing in the forward area it was never possible at any time to be sure that on the one hand only entirely suitable cases were returned to duty, and on the other that all cases sent to the base were necessitous.' W.G. MacPherson et al. (eds.), *History of the Great War*, p. 42. The same held true for members of the AIF.

21 Cooter, 'Malingering in Modernity: Psychological Scripts and Adversarial Encounters during the First World War', p.135.

22 Fuedtner, 'Minds the Dead Have Ravished', p. 396.

23 Unpublished work by J.W. Springthorpe: 'Australia at the War', MSS 755 AWM.

24 File: 14/8957. Case Papers (Australian Military Forces) 1915–1920. State Records of New South Wales.

25 File: 14/8959. State Records of New South Wales.

26 File: 14/8959. State Records of New South Wales.

27 File: 14/8958. State Records of New South Wales.

28 File: 14/8956. State Records of New South Wales.

29 File: 14/8956. State Records of New South Wales.

30 R. McMullin, *Pompey Elliott*, Scribe, Melbourne, 2002, p. 239.

31 J. Williams, *Anzacs, the Media and the Great War*, New South Wales University Press, 1999, p. 154.

32 Leese, *Shell Shock*, p. 26.

33 Letter to Butler from Dr John K. Adey (formerly lieutenant-colonel and commanding officer of the 5th Australian Field Ambulance and late Superintendent at the Royal Park Asylum, Melbourne) dated 20 April 1935. AWM 41 [280]. A similar observation was also made by Lieutenant-Colonel Walter Summons who thought it noteworthy that 'men with definite wounds are...far less liable to functional neuroses than those in whom no gross trauma has occurred.' W. Summons, 'Medical Work seen in the Australian Military Hospitals', *MJA*, 22 September 1917, p. 246.

34 Butler, *Official History*, vol. II, p. 59*n*.

35 Butler, *Official History*, vol. III, pp. 103–4.

36 Ibid., p. 102.

37 Leese, *Shell Shock*, p. 33.

38 Jones and Wessely, 'Psychiatric Battle Casualties: an Intra- and Interwar Comparison', pp. 242–3.

39 By 1916 French doctors such as Duprè and G. Roussy had espoused a 'chain' of events: commotion, èmotion, suggestion, exagèration, simulation and revendication (i.e. shock, emotion, suggestion, exaggeration, simulation and protesting).

40 J.W. Springthorpe, 'War Neuroses and Civil Practice', in *MJA*, 4 October 1919, p. 279. The Australian medical fraternity keenly followed developments in France. An early lesson was that based on the French model proposed by the *Societè Nèurologique*: 'expert neurologists should be engaged by the authorities to institute at an early date suitable treatment for soldiers suffering from these functional derangements, in order that they might be able to return to the firing-line as soon as possible.' Editorial: 'The Wastage from Incompleteness', *MJA*, 22 July 1916, p. 59.

41 P. Leese, 'Why are they not cured? British Shellshock Treatment During the Great War', in M. S. Micale and P. Lerner (eds.), *Traumatic Pasts: History, Psychiatry and Trauma in the Modern Age, 1870–1930*, Cambridge, 2001, p. 208.

42 Butler, *Official History*, vol. II, p. 462.

43 Summary by Colonel C.C. Manifold, DDMS Australian Corps 1 February 1918 to A.G. Butler. AWM 41 [659].

44 A.M. Wilson, A/ADMS, 'Moral and Mental Disorders—Shell Shock', 2nd Australian Division Report, undated c. 1918, p.1. AWM 41 /659.
45 File: 14/8956. State Records of New South Wales.
46 File: 14/8953. State Records of New South Wales.
47 File: 14/8956. State Records of New South Wales.
48 File: 14/8963. State Records of New South Wales.
49 File: 14/8953. State Records of New South Wales.
50 File: 14/8958. State Records of New South Wales.
51 For example in a hand-written note we see: 'The problem of the sub-normal (50 returned by the AIF). Not known to be deficient for some time...The country [Australia] should take responsibility of finding them employment.' C.E.W. Bean: 'Psychology: the Categories of Mentality', AWM 3 DRL 6673/530.
52 See C.E.W. Bean, 'The Battle of Pozieres, 1916', in *Official History of Australia in the War 1914–1918*, vol. III, p. 660.
53 Folder: 'Battle of Pozieres', AWM 3DRL 606.
54 C.E.W Bean, Diary 244, AWM 3DRL 606.
55 All these extracts are found in Bean's files, AWM 3DRL 606.
56 Diary of Corporal George R. Faulkner, stretcher bearer, 15th Australian Field Ambulance, France 1916, ML MSS 1151.
57 Damousi, *Freud*, p. 31.
58 Lance-Corporal A.J. Moore, stretcher bearer, 8th Australian Field Ambulance, ML MSS 911.
59 Private Longord Colley-Priest, diary, 19–22 July 1916, ML MSS 2439.
60 Sergeant W. C. Watson, 31st Battalion, France 1917, ML MSS 2949.
61 Diary written en route to Australia by Sapper Ernest De Mouncy, a signaller in the 4th Division, ML MSS 1839.
62 Report by Major C. B. Pym on a voyage from England to Australia aboard the HMT *Euripides*, September 1917. AWM 41 [280].
63 AWM 41 [280].
64 Springthorpe, 'Twelve Months' Service at the Front', p. 6.

Chapter Five
The Treatment of Shell Shock

It should be remembered that, during the First World War and for many decades afterwards, the condition of shell shock was poorly understood, and its treatment more so. As previously indicated the science of psychology was still in its infancy and even then its practitioners were divided amongst themselves. As a result, military doctors, especially those at the front, had little to work with but their own civilian experiences. Military officers found comfort in falling back onto the old disorders of empire including DAH or, worse, shrugging it off as cowardice. Nevertheless the war still saw earnest strides being taken to cure those who had succumbed to neuroses as a result of their experiences.

As both sides in the war fought themselves to exhaustion, the science of psychology evolved to meet the 'new' psychoses thrown up by this unprecedented cataclysm. Traditional medicine was seen as wanting—in providing both definitive treatment and even satisfactory explanations for these bizarre behaviours. While on the other side of the Atlantic American doctors proclaimed in 1918 that they had 'mastered' dealing with soldiers who were suffering from shell shock, even by 1919 it seemed that proponents of the 'new' ways of dealing with war neuroses had little to show for their efforts.[1] Lieutenant-Colonel J.W. Springthorpe (Senior Consultant Physician to the AIF) summed up the situation as an unfamiliar silence settled over the trenches: 'It is scarcely too much to say that, except in certain favoured spots, chaos brooded over the neurologically afflicted army and that, even yet, darkness remains over no small portion.'[2] It has also been said that shell shock 'threw into sharp relief the relationship between the mind and body, shell shock directly challenged earlier practices of diagnosing the mind.'[3] The various 'schools' of thought, which this encompassed will be dealt with later. For the moment though we will follow the soldier's progress through the evacuation chain from his initial trauma towards more 'definitive' care or, at least, reassessment. The lack of any sophistication attaching to the casualty's progress to a cure will be appreciated at once. As with wounds and sickness, the prime aim of psychiatric treatment of war neuroses was to return the soldier to active duty as soon as possible.

Hospital treatment for the hundreds of disturbed soldiers arriving in England in 1916 overwhelmed the few mental health facilities that had earlier been established for the military. Forward 'centres' for treating these men were then only just being established along the lines proposed earlier by the French. There was curiosity among commanders and military doctors as to their effectiveness. Were there many relapses amongst casualties treated close to the front? The historian is again dogged by lack of evidence, as one contemporary participant acknowledged: 'Unfortunately owing to the free movement of divisions from one army to another in accordance with varying military requirements, it is not possible to answer this with any accuracy.'[4] While statistics are absent, the influence of shell shock on all concerned and its stark contribution to the medical vocabulary was obvious to all. The official historian recorded that when shell shock became a generally recognised term, it was as if it were a new disease.

Consequently a 'complex terminology was evolved, and special treatments were manufactured in bewildering profusion. Some patients with hysterical symptoms were psycho-analysed, others with mental conflicts were hypnotized; whilst nearly all were treated on lines which could not fail to impress on the soldier's mind the mysteriousness of his malady.'[5] This is an accurate assessment of the medical confusion and the plethora of cures brought to bear on the problem of the neurotic soldier. But importantly the same confusion would drive soldiers who were otherwise sane but exhausted, into the arms of military medicine, convinced that they were indeed suffering from this new affliction.

Lieutenant-Colonel John Springthorpe was an 'old hand' at dealing with neuroses. Before joining the army he had been one of the earliest spokesmen for the mentally ill in Australia.[6] But even he was overwhelmed early in the war both by the numbers of casualties and the profusion of symptoms. Not unnaturally he sought advice from long-time colleague, Victoria's Inspector General for the Insane, Dr E. Jones. Writing to Jones about mentally ill soldiers being invalided to Australia in 1915 he asked 'if you would be good enough to make any suggestions or recommendations for the care of such cases.' Jones replied that the state would set aside the Royal Park Receiving House in Melbourne and that he could 'see no reason at all why the other States in Australia should not fall into line.'[7] Ultimately this is what occurred, although it was not unusual for a man's relatives to care for him at home if the authorities considered this to be in the patient's best interest and that he posed no threat of violence.

In retrospect it is perhaps surprising that so many soldiers at that time recovered from their neuroses. Colonel Sir Harry Maudsley who was the AIF's senior consulting psychologist was content to classify war neuroses into two categories

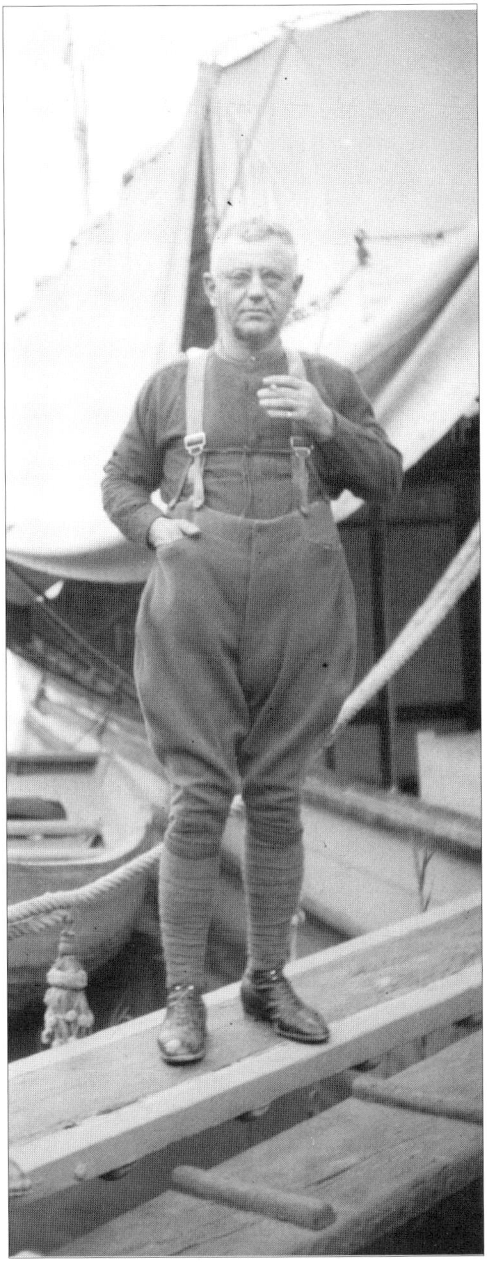

Lieutenant-Colonel J.W. Springthorpe. c.1917. (AWM PS1087 – image enhanced by the author)

that he referred to as 'Conversion Hysterics' and 'Anxiety States' or men suffering from neurasthenia. He wrote that he had seen many war neurotics admitted to hospitals. 'They had been afflicted for months and had been under treatment in British hospitals and in our own auxiliary hospitals. It is evident that most of them were permanently unfit for general service; a small minority might be fit after six months' rest.' Still, he was optimistic and thought that most of these casualties would be fit for duty 'away from the front, or in civil life' in a matter of months.[8] However, a percentage of the traumatised would never recover. These men were true psychotic cases and upon their return to Australia they would be admitted (albeit without the stigma of being 'certified' in recognition of their war service) to one of the few military asylums or to the wider civilian asylum system. But closer to the front confusion remained.

One of the first problems encountered concerned the fact that early in the war many soldiers admitted to military or civilian asylums or specialist medical centres should never have been there. Bearing in mind the sometimes transitory and often confused effects of shell shock on the individual, medical officers not unnaturally erred on the side of caution when diagnosing casualties. During the war there was a bewildering range of medical indicators for neurotic soldiers. In addition to the increasing, if illicit use of the term 'shell shock' popular amongst the soldiers themselves and the folk at home, the list included 'Effort Syndrome'; DAH; GPI (General Paralysis of Insane); NYDN—Not Yet Diagnosed

(Nervous); NYDN (W)—shell shock with wound; and NYDN (S)—shell shock, no wound.[9] Once the use of the terms 'shell shock W[ounded]' and 'shell shock' were officially proscribed as a diagnosis in the army in 1917, NYDN became the new catch-all rubric, perhaps not in a way dissimilar to the PTSD well known in our own age.

Whereas one medical officer might have diagnosed a soldier as suffering from 'shell shock', to another doctor the same man may have appeared as simply overwrought or even simply depressed. For those affected, shell shock was an intensely personal psychological experience. The problem of empiricism in battle stress remains today, despite the huge advances made in psychology and neurological sciences since 1918. What is stress? Some have defined it as 'the physiological and psychological reaction that occurs when individuals perceive an imbalance between the level of demand placed on them and their capacity to meet that demand. Individuals experience stress as an internal, personal response that cannot be measured by onlookers.'[10] But while the experience was mentally 'internal' it was quickly obvious to a soldier's mates when he was becoming neurotic or was shocked after being buried or blown up by an artillery shell. Like other commonplaces on the battlefield these situations fell into the popular slang of the soldiery—'losing his nut', 'dotty', 'queer' and 'loony'.

The situation at the front was worse during times of heavy fighting when sheer numbers overwhelmed doctors and their primitive dressing stations. This precluded any detailed triage or assessment of soldiers who, in some instances, were only momentarily stunned. Of course the war demanded nothing less than a total effort and everything in the military's meagre medical arsenal was thrown at the problem of shell shock. A. G. Butler wrote that 'in this and other matters the war situation required *results*.' Besides the basic principles of rest, sleep, food, quiet and so forth, experts tried 'hypnotism, suggestion, persuasion, stimulation and discipline.' He added without irony that 'deep analysis' techniques usually left to specialists were not used at the front.[11]

So the numbers of 'true' neuroses being evacuated to hospitals as far back as London were probably inflated by soldiers who just needed reassurance and respite from the trying conditions of often fruitless offensive operations or 'stunts' at the front. Basic triage or sorting of casualties also would have identified those suffering from psychoses (generally regarded as more serious if not intractable) and those suffering from neuroses. A British practitioner described the processing of the shell-shocked soldier as it worked in 1916: 'On arrival at one of the British base hospitals abroad the soldier's condition is investigated by a special medical officer. The patient is then sent to a section of the hospital according as his symptoms are of a neurological or a mental character. Should he be suffering from transitory mental symptoms, which subside rapidly, he is transferred from the mental to the neurological section as soon as it is advisable to do so.'[12]

Many doctors with experience in civilian asylums had joined the AAMC and it was this group that now managed mental cases in the medical infrastructure that was growing to cope with these soldiers' suffering. It was to be expected that doctors would bring their own pet theories and prejudices along with them, although this did not always work in their patients' favour. 'Since neither psychiatrists nor physicians were trained analysts, it is not surprising that the practice of psychoanalysis would be a major point of dispute, and that many of Freud's ideas were adopted eclectically.'[13] However, be they civil or military, 'alienists' or psychological specialists were all drawn from the existing mental health system.

A number of British alienists were associated with the public asylum system, a practice mirrored in Australia. 'The psychological interpretations and treatments of shell shock developed largely within the English military mental hospitals. These institutions promoted a new wartime social arrangement between mental patients and physicians, one strikingly different from that of the asylum setting.'[14] Some of these centres would develop into teaching hospitals and significant centres for psychological research. In the case of Australian troops who were treated under this system, the Red Cross Military Hospital at Maghull near Liverpool, the Seale Hayne Neurological Hospital (under Lieutenant-Colonel Arthur Hurst) in Devon and the No. 3 Australian Auxiliary Hospital at Dartford were the most important.[15] The concentration of Australian psychiatric casualties in just a few select centres was the deliberate policy of the Australian Army, which was concerned not to lose its authority or national identity within the vast British system.[16] But other hospitals played a significant part in this side of the war's medical history, the better known of these institutions including the Royal Victoria Military Hospital at Netley, Napsbury War Hospital, and Queen's Square. As we shall see, it was at these centres that the new disciples of psychology sought to weave their own notions of magic.

The concept of treating soldiers for shell shock and neuroses closer to the front line was not taken up by the British until quite late in the war, although some AAMC officers (including the influential ex-Indian Army officer Colonel C. C. Manifold who had been seconded to the AIF) were strong proponents of such a strategy. Not until late 1917 did Australian medical units begin systematically to treat soldiers at the front. A senior Australian medical officer wrote that care was being taken that 'slight cases of nerve exhaustion' were retained at Advanced and Main Dressing Stations where they were rested, given food and returned to their unit for duty. He was forced to admit, however, that some of these casualties 'will be found to be incapable of carrying on in the face of shellfire.' In a rare statement for an official, he also admitted what many doctors suspected: that 'no doubt in the past many of these cases have been labelled "coward" wrongfully as often it is entirely a matter of environment and circumstances.'[17]

The French, on the other hand (and admittedly the war was on their soil), took a different approach which involved more immediate medical intervention.[18] As early as October 1915, Centres Neurologiques Règionaux had been established throughout the country, later augmented in April 1916 by Centres Neurologiques d'Armeès which were sited at key areas of troop concentrations in the evacuation chain and were staffed by specialists. Springthorpe reported on one of his inspection visits that the French divided their war neuroses into several categories. These were: 'functional', 'Neuro-psychiatrique-Commotionel-Emotionel', and 'organic'. He visited several clinics, including that of Dr Babinksi at Le Pitiè and Briand's clinic at Val de Grâce.[19] The location of such 'clinics' close to the front seemed to provide an answer.[20] 'Andrè Lèri, working in the centre attached to the French Second Army, reported that '91% of admissions between July and October 1916 were returned to the fighting line.'[21]

As the manpower wastage from illness grew, the military had to take more draconian steps and the method of dealing with neuroses changed. This example is just one of the five circulars issued between January and March 1917 to Australian army medical units: 'The DDMS directs that no cases classified as "shell shock" or nervous (breakdown, inability to stand shellfire and neurasthenia) are to be evacuated to Field Ambulances unless very definite symptoms are present. Cases of fright and hysteria are to be retained and treated in the lines.'[22] In fact no case was to be evacuated from the divisional area until he was seen *personally* by the Acting Deputy or Deputy Director of Medical Services, a very high ranking officer.

In Germany, which had seen significant advances in the understanding and treatment of mental illness, a different approach was sometimes taken. As the war unfolded the attitude increasingly mirrored that country's psychiatrists' concept of the war 'as a giant industrial accident, and from the war's early phases [they] approached neurotic soldiers like injured industrial workers.'[23] This thinking would come to the British much later, as it would, to a lesser extent, to the Australians. But in both Germany and Austria, by early 1915 psychoanalysts had been brought in 'to treat Kreigsneurotiker.'[24] There were long-standing formal links between psychologists and the army that dated back to 1890. These men had been engaged in refining recruiting methods on behalf of the German military. One of Germany's luminaries in this field, Emil Kraepelin, had collaborated closely with the Bavarian War Ministry since 1905.[25] Some German and Austrian army practitioners looked at the problem in a different light to their British and French opponents. 'In fact, rather than blaming the shocks and stresses of the battlefield for the onset of war neuroses, many [German] psychiatrists began to see war as a kind of cure, as a moral and psychological corrective to a civil society they deemed effeminate, degenerate and pathogenic.'[26] The war was to be a sort mental cleansing of the weaker vessels of the state.

Germany was subject not only to increasing censorship of intellectual debate but it also saw a swing away from a predominantly sympathetic school of psychiatric care (exemplified by Doctor Hermann Oppenheim), to the views shared with the British school of industrial compensation (with its propensity for suspicion) and with the eugenics movement. Subsequently many German treatment regimes were severe.[27] But then the same could be said of England as some scholars have revealed. Psychology came to treat neurasthenia 'as though it were a disease of the "will", rather than of "nerve force".' This had important ramifications for the mentally ill because, in a bizarre twist of military logic, it made these stricken men increasingly blameworthy for their own illnesses. 'Conventional cures stressing the need for rest were jettisoned on the grounds that they could encourage laziness—ultimately destructive of manliness.'[28]

Those, like Freud, who used psychological trauma to explain shell shock, were effectively sidestepped by a state with its eyes fixed not only on a total military victory, but on husbanding human and financial resources to ensure this outcome. 'The harsh treatment of those who suffered from shell-shock was meant to cure men of their weakness and send them back to the front.'[29] Hermann Oppenheim, the Berlin neurologist, was a significant personality in prewar German psychology and an early proponent of the traumatic neurosis diagnosis approach 'which treated post-traumatic nervous symptoms as a distinct entity resulting from the direct—anatomical or psychic—effects of traumatic events.' Like Frederick (later Sir Frederick) Mott in Britain, he initially supported the organic, rather than the psychological approach to shell shock. But, unfortunately, once the war began, his star waned because his diagnosis of shell-shocked soldiers would have 'guaranteed' them pensions. He was therefore 'condemned for "artificially creating" epidemics of neurosis and the idea was generally seen as scientifically false.'[30] And so, as in England, the military authorities won the day to the detriment of many traumatised soldiers.

Treatment regimes within the British and Australian military encompassed the full suite of psychological theories and schools of thought then in vogue. Popular hospital treatment included rest, quiet rooms, individual rooms, darkened rooms, milk diets, physiotherapy, army drill, psychotherapy by means of hypnosis or 'suggestion', individual 'counselling with alienists or doctors', hot and cold showers, electric shock, fresh air, outdoor work, gardening, furniture making, hobbies and spas. However not everyone agreed with what some regarded as mollycoddling the patient. 'War shock requires vigorous treatment and return to active life as soon as possible. The reckless way in which a rest cure and overfeeding are ordered indiscriminately for all persons suffering from any form of psycho-neurosis reveals lamentable ignorance.' This doctor believed that suggestion and psychoanalysis was 'the most fruitful method of treatment in war-shock.'[31] In one Australian hospital, patients were not allowed to consider themselves invalids. Instead they were roused from their beds early in the morning by a barking sergeant-major, given fatigues (usually tedious tasks), placed on the parade ground for military drill and taken on route marches. Where these soldiers had a trade they were put to work. Even here, however, there were some, 'particularly recurrent cases, whom it is probably unwise to send back to the line although in good physical condition, but if discrimination is exercised here, much of the potent value of the Centre will be destroyed.'[32]

The main types of treatment to which a shell-shocked soldier might find himself subjected were many and varied. But there was generally a core of well tried, if not tested, techniques. 'Persuasion', a favourite of Dr W. R. Regnell, was used by medical officers, sometimes with moral blackmail (letting down mates etc.) or even threats, to get the soldier back in the trenches. Other doctors used 'explanation' in which the patient was told that he was not suffering from any irreversible or mysterious illness but 'could be cured with his cooperation.' 'Expression' was another favoured technique. 'The psychotherapists at Maghull and Netley developed an approach to the treatment of shell shock based on various "abreactive" or "cathartic" techniques designed to get patients to re-live and re-experience painful "emotional memories" which had been buried from consciousness.'[33] Some practitioners claimed a high success rate with this method.

'Suggestion' was often used to bluff the patient into thinking he was curing himself and that his normal functions were actually resuming. This was often assisted by hypnosis, as espoused by Charles Myers. Another method was 're-education' in which the soldier's sense of duty was 're-awakened' 'through propagandising him in the military and social necessities.' Lastly there was the outdoors school (to which Butler and Bean subscribed); that is, fresh air, gardening or other work outdoors during daylight hours as a way of getting soldiers to come to terms with their experiences. What happened when the dark and solitude of night enveloped them is not mentioned. Freudian psychoanalysis was, according to A. G. Butler, a 'closed cult', but he had to admit that the 'essential principles and concepts of Freudian psychology 'were indeed an essential part of the stock-in-trade of the officers who from early 1917 were responsible' for psychiatric cases at the front.[34] Other practitioners preferred a 'simpler and more direct procedure' than Freudian analysis— abreaction. According to Queenslander Dr J. P. Lowson, this method, which he had used on 'war neurotics', aimed at 'clearing up a single incident' in the life of the victim, and not, as was the case in analysis, at solving all his principal emotional needs.[35]

Generally, throughout the military, suspected cases of malingering were dealt with through isolation, dietary restrictions, confinement and disciplinary measures. In February 1918 Colonel C. C. Manifold was to write of the need for 'necessary disciplinary firmness' to be exercised by medical officers, especially at the front. 'There was certainly one glaring instance of this in a battalion in which the OC [Officer Commanding], to stop the rot caused by such mistaken weakness, had to ask that the RMO might be removed. This, of course, was a very exceptional case.'[36] This view was not universally shared, however. Even after the war, Dr D. M. McWhae, himself a former medical officer, admitted that, while there was a place for hypnosis in treatment, he still believed that '...firmness, persistence and kindness will in the end succeed in removing the hysterical victim in the vast majority of cases.'[37] Even the relatively non-invasive method of hypnosis with an often quite successful record of cures was, with its 'savour of the uncanny, the mysterious and the unknown', frowned upon by the military. Others believed that hypnosis could only work with the weak-minded.[38]

In Britain, the army's senior psychologist, Lieutenant-Colonel Charles Myers, also dismissed the malingerer theory outright and, in referring to his own patients, concluded that despite 'the slow progress', he had not the slightest doubt that hypnosis 'invariably proved of great assistance towards recovery.' He added that it would have been of even greater value 'if it could have been occasionally repeated later.'[39] In the medical profession itself there was a hint of bitterness even in legitimate examples of neurosis. One Australian medical officer, in looking back over the war, included this piqued observation in a 1918 report:

> Many of us remember well the numbers of cases labelled 'shell shock–wounded' coming through the stations during the early part of the Somme Offensive. All these men were classed as battle-casualties and many of these men are wearing gold wound stripes; whereas their comrades who saw the battle out have no reward except their own personal satisfaction.[40]

The policy of the shell shock centre established at No. 2 AGH in France was unequivocal. It was to 'secure the return of all possible cases to their units; it is therefore allowed to be understood among patients that they will return to the front as soon as fit, without alternative and that evacuation to England or transfer to base units will not be considered.'[41] This foreshadowed developments twenty years later when 'the principles of proximity, expectancy and immediacy' became a maxim of military psychology. Under this method the victim could 'get the rest that is the only current cure for his problem, while not giving a message to his healthy comrades that insanity is a ticket away from the madness of the battlefield.'[42]

Others were more compassionate (and therefore made poor army officers according to the old school of military hardliners). A psychology authority wrote that soldiers suffering from shell shock were as suitable for return to fighting as were their physically wounded counterparts. He recommended that after a 'cure' had been effected, these men should be 'sent forthwith to the Front. Six weeks to three months after cure is required, the first part of which time I cannot think but might be spent on furlough with his family; the latter part in one of the convalescent camps where the soldier will be gradually retrained.'[43]

A 1917 report sent by Lieutenant-Colonel J.W. Springthorpe to the Deputy Director of Medical Services provides some insight not only into the overall management of the shell-shocked soldier by that stage of the war, but also into what was actually happening in military attitudes to shell shock—physiologically and psychologically. First, the author attempted to classify 'neurological war cases' albeit still attributing shell shock itself to physical or organic causes. [44] These categories were:

a) Organic—with recognised lesions and localisations [sic],
b) Neurasthenic—from physical and mental exhaustion following strain,
c) Psychological—predominantly mental,
d) Hysteroid—with persistent auto-suggestion,
e) Hyperthyroid—Hyper-adrenal exaggerated defensive reflexes etc., and
f) Shell Shock—due to high explosives of various kinds.

He then proceeded to describe causes and symptoms as well as preventative measures. Then, with a faint allusion to hysteria, he described the cause of shell shock as a 'sudden over whelming concussion generally combined with concentrated emotional overthrow.' When first seen by the RMO, the patient was often dazed or unconscious (sometimes for weeks), 'in others instantly killed without any sign of external injury.' These variations in 'confusion, dullness, concentration, excitability and depression, with giddy turns and defects of memory, up to complete amnesia may persist for months or even years.' Sleep was usually limited and the patient restless, while his immediate past 'often recurs nightly in more or less terrifying dreams.' Springthorpe, one of the increasing numbers of doctors who actually *listened* to these men, also described vertigo, constant headaches and tremors in the soldiers presenting at medical aid posts.[45] The best way to treat these men was, according to Springthorpe, in 'a favourable environment, sufficient rest, special feeding, suitable influences and suggestions, and graduated exercise of mind and body.' He also believed that there would be fewer and less dramatic cases if recruits 'were carefully selected, individually placed and trained and frequently rested.'[46]

As the war progressed and observers now had the time to assimilate ideas from better informed clinical meetings and the medical literature, and could see for themselves what seemed to work and what didn't, various views crystallised into specific programs. By 1917 Springthorpe was alive to the possibilities that presented themselves for a cure when patients were allowed to mix and interact freely in the civilian world. Consequently he had established a network of sympathetic English families who were happy to host his hospital patients, take them on outings or even keep them in their own homes for short periods. However an unyielding military bureaucracy put a stop to this enlightened approach. Frustrated he wrote to the commanding officer of the special Australian hospital at Dartford asking him to explain why no sick leave could be granted to this category of patient. 'I have continuously and repeatedly made use of sick leave for selected "shell shock" patients both to satisfactory friends and relatives and, in the case of the friendless, to approved English homes ever since I took charge of such cases last November.'[47] In a minute dated 27 August 1917, the Director of Australia's Medical Services, an over-worked Major-General Neville Howse VC, wrote that 'after due consideration and discussion of the matter, there do not appear to be sufficient reasons for departing from the order that no leave is to be granted.'

By 1916 the AAMC offered three-month specialist courses in neurasthenic work (including 'abreactive' techniques) to its own medical officers and those of the Empire and its allies. This training was organised at the Red Cross Military Hospital, Maghull. While American and Canadian officers attended, AAMC officers were refused permission to attend by Major-General Howse, presumably because the small Australian Corps could not spare them from more urgent duties. However he did advise the AAMC in England that a series 'of lectures on matters of neurological interest will shortly be delivered by Colonel Mott [who still subscribed to the organic theory], Neurologist at Maudsley Neurological Hospital.'[48] If any medical officers wished to attend the lectures then arrangements could be made for them to do so. It seems that whatever form of training was attended later paid dividends. Early in 1919 Colonel D. M. McWhae, the ADMS for the AIF's depots in the UK, sent a memorandum to all his officers there informing them that, since Major J. B. Lewis had returned from 'the School of Neurology at Seale Hayne Hospital, all Australian soldiers suffering from 15 separate conditions ranging from mutism to incontinence were to go before this officer for a medical examination.'[49]

In much of the (English language) literature about shell shock, emphasis is often placed on the socio-economic class of the neurotic soldier as a means not only of explaining the different reactions to mental trauma, but also subsequent treatment regimes and public attitudes to the plight of these men. 'The class distinction drawn by psychological theories between treatment for officers and men—intelligent hobbies v. useful work—was another attribute of the psychological perspective. The superior social position of the officers demanded that they be treated in accordance with their more "refined" and educated class.'[50] In discussions of the medical evacuation chain for mental cases, it has also been stated that inevitably the place of an individual case within that gradation of therapeutic strategies 'was heavily dependent on social status.'[51] Within the Australian context, however, much of this comment is simply inappropriate.

While it is simplistic to suggest that there were no class barriers in early twentieth century Australia, the composition of the largely voluntary AIF did not share the hidebound distinctions that characterised the British Army system. Even Kitchener's more 'democratic' New Army could hardly ignore long-ingrained social mores and expectations. These class prejudices extended to the medical profession as well and Australian doctors (in their postwar correspondence) do occasionally speak of an officer 'group' if not of a 'class.' This said, one still finds references to class as a psychological indicator in the Australian medical literature as late as 1930. Explaining how officers had tended to develop neurasthenia while private soldiers presented with (the more demeaning) hysteria, Dr Roy Winn, a psychologist himself, wrote that the difference was due to education which 'leads to the more complete integration of the personality by favouring development of the self-regarding [esteem] sentiment.'[52]

Early in the war, shell shock, at least in Britain, was regarded as typifying the inherent weakness of the working class soldier. It had yet to make any inroads on the newly arriving Australians. In contrast, nervous breakdowns by officers were often regarded more sympathetically and excused more often on the basis of the officer's sensibility and refinement. However as the war progressed and more and more officers from non-traditional backgrounds came forward to fill the diminishing ranks of what had been the strict preserve of the Edwardian 'gentleman', excuses for breakdown amongst these parvenus still had to be explained away and the old resort to class superiority now sounded hollow. There are parallels with the AIF, if not concerning the place of class in the issue of war neuroses, then in the distinction between officers and men in the casualty figures. In the British Army 'in a 1918 sample of officers only six per cent were sent back to duty, whereas 66 per cent were sent back to the base camp. By contrast, among lower ranks, 27 per cent were sent straight back to duty, and only 36 per cent were sent to the base camp...Inevitably the place of an individual within that gradation was heavily dependent on social status.'[53] This observation also says more of the higher utility value (as canon-fodder) of the private soldier than the officer.

Conversely, too much can be made of the egalitarian aspect of the Australian military at the time. This, together with the ambiguity of diagnosis and the paucity of reliable statistics, makes some claims less reliable than they seem and they should therefore be regarded with caution. One writer has claimed that Australian doctors 'consistently' reported fewer cases of shell shock compared with British figures. During the fighting around Pozières in 1916 'when the British figure was nearing 40 per cent, Australian doctors estimated that only one-quarter of ordinary soldiers, and even fewer officers treated were suffering from shell-shock.' He went on to suggest that 'the renowned "mateship" of the Anzacs may have acted as a psychological bulwark against shell shock, reducing its prevalence.'[54] This is an over-simplification, given that similar bonds held together British and French units, particularly 'old' regiments, just as effectively. It is now known that close unit cohesion and high morale is an effective antidote for some neuroses on the battlefield. The statement also contradicts anecdotal evidence and the known propensity of medical officers at this time to shield officers particularly from the aspersions associated with shell shock.

Within this complex system of hospitals, mental and general, field ambulances, and specialist centres, men—the genuinely neurotic and the rest—were sometimes shuttled about at random, as unsure of themselves as the doctors were of their condition. They might receive a variety of treatments, some of them antagonistic, others cancelling any gains made by their predecessors. There was confusion and, given the chaos and demands of wartime, this situation more or less survived to 1919. So, by war's end, in 'the area of aetiology of war neurosis...a form of stalemate had emerged.'[55]

Halfway through 1917 the authorities not only prescribed the use of the phrase 'shell shock' as a diagnostic label, they also tried to introduce more certainty into this fraught area by means of a bureaucratic solution. This took the shape of a field medical questionnaire or card—the ubiquitous *Form AF 3436*—the administration of which turned out to be unworkable. At this time Australian medical officers at the front were still more or less left to their own devices when it came to diagnosis. Early in the war there was little in the way of scientific psychological literature or clinical education in the field. Some have seen more sinister motives behind this. 'Shell-shock then was so obviously a retreat from the war that the British military tried to keep it from the public: when Myers requested permission in 1916 to publish a book on the features and causation of shell-shock, he was told that the General Staff strongly opposed any such publication.'[56] After all, it was embarrassing for the War Office and the AIF to admit that hundreds of its soldiers were succumbing to mental breakdowns or worse, hysteria.

However the War Office did not seem to mind burdening its medical system by introducing more paperwork and delay. It has been suggested (not without evidence) that because of the British Adjutant-General's distrust of doctors, no shell-shocked man 'could receive...specialist attention until *Form AF 3436* had been sent off to the man's unit and filled in by his commanding officer.'[57] Much time was wasted in this Kafkaesque paper labyrinth. In November that year Springthorpe had trialled a similar 'neurosis card' to facilitate ongoing treatment. The instructions contained in it for RMOs reflect his own ambiguity to shell shock. Doctors were told to fill in the card after 'the elimination of (1) organic brain conditions of any kind (2) the mentally and physically sound but temporarily "knocked out", and (3) the malingerers, in whom "the party's criminal will" feigns symptoms that do not exist.'[58] The first question was: 'In the family there has been: hysteria, epilepsy, insanity, neurasthenia, nervous breakdown, nervous instability?'

While on an inspection of AAMC units in Europe in 1918, the Corps' second most senior officer, Major-General Richard Fetherston, reported his views on the treatment of Australian soldiers in two military hospitals he visited in Britain. Much of what he saw there was 'very far ahead of anything so far attempted in Australia.' The first establishment was the Golders Green Hospital of Shell Shock, Neurasthenia and Allied Conditions. Most of its patients were 'shell shock cases with a large hysterical element. There are a large number of neurasthenics—a chronic condition in many cases—present to a large extent before enlistment, and these cases are difficult to improve.' Like many treatment regimes, emphasis was placed on occupational therapy such as gardening. Fetherston picked up on what most officers there must have discussed with him and that concerned the delay in their patients' treatment—of whatever kind—between their 'wounding' and being admitted to a large-scale medical facility. This, they suggested, had delayed a cure. Fetherston also reported that, for the previous two years, many Australian patients had apparently received 'very little active treatment in the military hospitals and the condition has been allowed to drag on and no rational or intensive treatment has been applied for months after it might have been commenced.' While this says more of the hopelessly understaffed specialist hospitals' ability to cope with their workload, it may also explain why so many 'relapses' were seen in these patients years after the war.

Fetherston then spoke of the 300-bed Seale Hayne Hospital at Newton Abbot (near Torquay) where no 'hypnotic or electrical treatment is given nor are drugs used, reliance being placed on intense moral persuasion and encouragement.' But here the approach was different. He noted that doctors 'might remain with one patient from half to three hours at one sitting' while 'electricity and massage have been practically discarded, and hypnotism except for rare cases.' In both establishments most of the patients were 'cases of functional disease, hysterical paralysis, paraplegia, aphonias etc. and had never been under shell fire at all.' He concluded his report with reference to contemporary orthodoxy by calling attention to the 'fact that a large proportion of the so-called cases of shell shock are really cases of nervous breakdown under the stress of war in patients predisposed by mental instability...'[59]

One Australian doctor working at Newton Abbot in 1918 optimistically reported that 'we made it a rule to keep a man in hospital until he was fit to return to duty or direct to his civilian occupation. Of patients discharged from the service very few, indeed, needed a pension at all [then], but many of them were given one of 20% or less.'[60] Another Australian, A. E. Rowden White, later reported his experiences in a smaller hospital in Oxford. There, each medical officer had his own special way of dealing with patients, but would adopt *any* plan shown by his colleagues to be of use. There is more than a hint of desperation in his comment: 'Analysis was carried out either while the patient was awake (psychoanalysis) or during induced sleep (hypnoanalysis).' He cautioned that 'much harm was done by allowing charlatans to persuade the public that they alone could carry out this treatment.'[61] It remains unclear to what extent his comment was due to professional parochialism or real fear of incompetent treatment.

In contrast to Britain where the government had no option but to let servicemen return immediately to their families, Australian soldiers often had to wait up to a year before they saw home. How much this enforced period with their mates in formed units assisted a complete recovery will never be known, but the opportunity for long 'yarns', informal debriefings and talks between friends, often of the same unit, must have been cathartic. From mid-1917 mental patients were repatriated where possible in transport ships allocated specially for them, rather than mixing them with the bulk of the returning army.[62] A specialist medical officer accompanied these men, together with orderlies who were often selected on the basis of their previous experience working in asylums. Where lack of shipping did not allow separate vessels, part of the troop-ship would be screened off for psychiatric soldiers. A sophisticated evacuation system evolved. 'The Mental Unit (No. 10 Sea Transport Section, AAMC, AIF) was made up as follows: 1 medical officer, one warrant officer (ward master), one staff sergeant dispenser; three sergeants; three corporals and 24 privates.' Butler records that from June 1917 'some 300 mental invalids (apart from minor psychoses—"shell shocks") were sent in this manner with great advantage to the patients themselves.'[63]

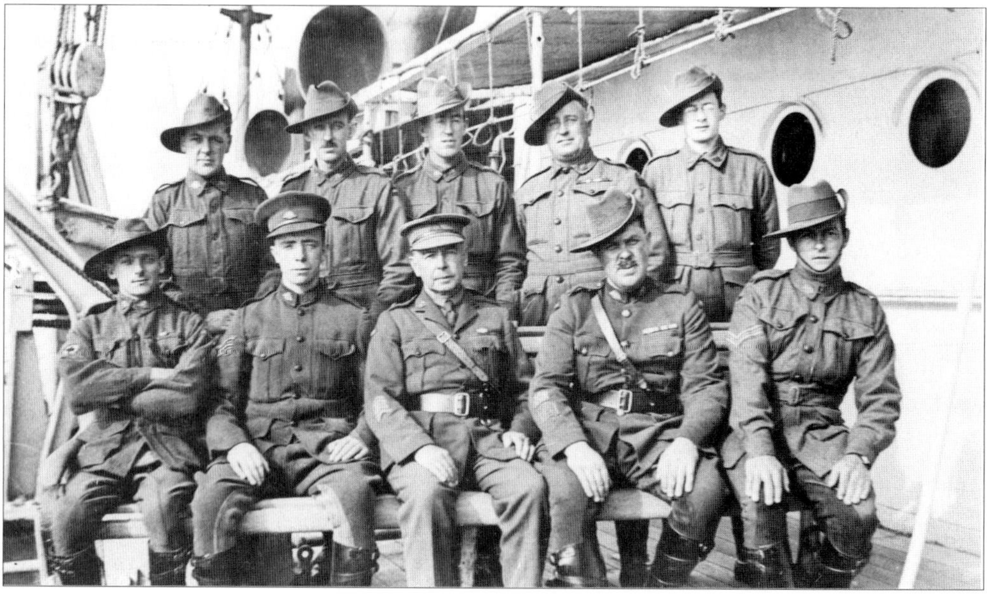

Major C.B. Pym (second from the right, front row) and members of the No.10 Sea Transport Section on board the troop-ship *Borda*.
(AWM H18930)

'Home' and the expectation of a return were identified by some Australian medical officers as playing an important role in the progress of mental patients. In February 1919 Colonel D. McWhae wrote an extensive report for Australian authorities. In it he admitted that the treatment of war neuroses at the AIF's main depot at Weymouth in England had been 'extremely difficult to deal with during active hostilities. Despite intensive re-education the counter suggestion induced by the knowledge that men would possibly have to return to France if they were cured greatly effected [sic] the results of treatment.' However of those patients repatriated to Australia many 'improved rapidly while under treatment of the voyage.' Like most of his colleagues, McWhae had not seen home or family since 1915 and could only guess what the situation was like there when it came to dealing with the psychological detritus of the war. He assumed however, that there 'must be a large number of soldiers with war neuroses in Australia, either still under treatment or discharged as pensioners.' His own experience had shown him the importance of such men being assessed by suitably trained doctors, or by Australian officers who had had the chance to attend specialist courses or be seconded to British institutions such as the Seale Hayne and other hospitals. He had seen hundreds of war neurotics who had received inadequate advice or treatment, or who 'had never been told that any treatment could help them.' His message home was clear—'there must be a large number of discharged soldiers in Australia drawing pensions who are suffering from war neuroses which are entirely curable.'[64]

The *Medical Journal of Australia* reported on a seminal medical conference for senior officers of the AAMC held on 17 June 1918 in Melbourne. They had determined to employ the term 'neurasthenia' to include 'ordinary neurasthenia and hysteria as seen in civil practice'; 'shell shock'; debility associated with well-marked toxic or functional disorders of the nervous system, 'such as is observed under the rubric of "disordered action of the heart"; and thyro-toxic disturbances.' They also decided that patients suffering from neurasthenia should not be granted 'boat leave', but 'should be admitted direct from the hospital ship or hospital transport to the military hospital, for the purposes of observation and treatment.'[65]

As the flow of shell-shocked diggers began to reach Australia, a system similar to that operating in England was instigated. The military decided to use both the extant civilian asylum system (better funded and staffed than its British counterpart which was still linked to the antiquated Poor Laws), supplemented by a small amount of specialist military accommodation. Often these were large mansions taken over for the war effort and with the stroke of a pen transformed into the seemingly grand 'Australian Auxiliary Hospitals' (AAH). The commanding officer of one such establishment provided a brief history of his establishment—Broughton Hall in Sydney. This hospital was opened in 1915 (in a deteriorating house originally built in 1842) to accommodate fifty patients in a rented property. A 1917 report stated that most of these men suffered from 'minor psychopathies' and that they recovered after an 'appropriate' course of treatment. Insane and 'troublesome' cases were placed in a detached cottage in the spacious garden surroundings of the Callan Park Mental Hospital across the street. The 'overflow' was sent to the asylum proper. During 1917 additions were made to the military 'cottage', increasing the number of beds from nine to twenty-five. 'Of 241 admissions to Broughton Hall between 1915 and 1917, 160 were discharged (of whom 20 were classed "non-recovered or relieved").'[66]

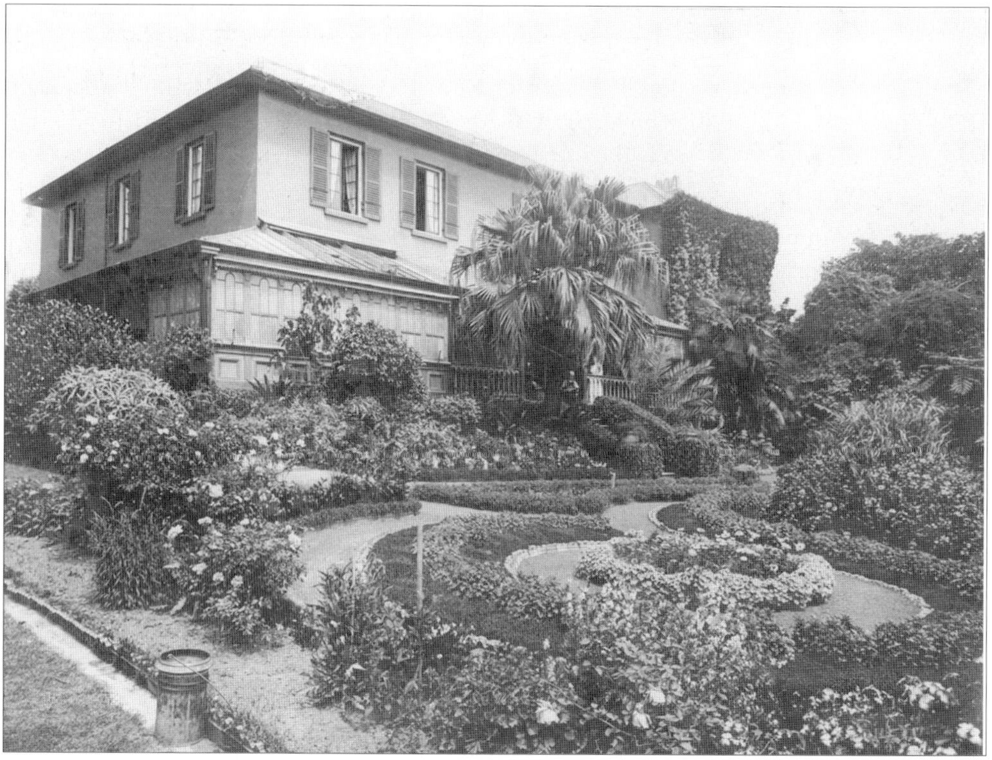

Broughton Hall, a privately owned mansion at the turn of the nineteenth century. Its lush gardens provided an oasis for soldiers sent there to 'recover' from their psychiatric problems. (Friends of Callan Park, Sydney)

Shell shock had also gripped the popular imagination, its images particularly stark in a civilian population that had little concept of the realities of trench warfare. In 1916, at what was a relatively early stage of the war, and long before the trauma of the fighting around Pozières, *The Times Illustrated History of the War* attempted to explain to the layperson in non-clinical terms what shell shock was, its cause and how it affected soldiers.[67] The relevant chapter was also illustrated with photographs of various pieces of equipment and men undergoing mental rehabilitation. Public education such as this could only cement the sympathy already felt by the person in the street towards the mental wrecks that were now a feature of casualty disembarkations in England at ports and railway stations all around the country.

While in Australia there was nothing comparable to the *Times* article, the Australian public too was quick to take these men to their hearts. As we shall see, however, this community sympathy proved to be fickle and diminished after the war to be replaced by antipathy among the non ex-service community during the 1920s and 1930s. Others found the publicity unwelcome, seeing it as a medium of contagion. A senior Australian medical officer suggested that 'there were other factors to be considered besides those of the men being under new and severe conditions of fire.' He was referring to the popular press coverage of shell shock and the fact that 'there was almost a tendency to regard it as a Society Doctor's patients might a new fashionable complaint.'[68]

It was not all gloom and doom however, and it would be wrong to assume that *all* soldiers who suffered psychological problems ended up as chronic sufferers. There were hundreds of cases at individual institutions in which soldiers were treated successfully and in periods sometimes measured as short as minutes. Conditions including aphonia, stammering and 'psycoasthenia' were cured by suggestion.[69] A major hurdle for these patients which often prevented their being admitted in the first place was the lack of understanding by front-line RMOs (through no fault of theirs) of the cause and management of these manifestations of shell shock. Time and overwhelming casualty numbers were ever the medical officers' enemies at the front. There is also no doubt that individual commanders at divisional, regimental and battalion levels all had their own prejudices and understanding of 'shell shock' and how it should be treated. As a result, soldiers continued to face the twin challenges of predisposition from the medical fraternity and malingering from the military command.

On 31 March 1921 the AIF, except for a few troops and specialist officers still left overseas, officially ceased to exist, and the whole responsibility for treatment of war disabilities now came to rest with the Department of Repatriation.[70] This worked to the advantage of a mentally damaged soldier as it meant a concerted, if not always coordinated, approach to his problems and a genuine attempt to do the best by him as far as the army, his pension entitlements and his medical treatment were concerned. But for many it would be a difficult return to the society they had left years previously —a society which had moved on, as they themselves had done.

Describing a 26-year-old corporal whose three brothers had already been killed in the war and who had been subjected to a shell burst at Messines in June 1917, Major Archie Fraser recounted his care for this patient on the long sea voyage home. In his notes he records a common anxiety felt by those on their way back to Australia, sometimes after an absence of four years. 'He was not worried by the memory of battle scenes, he did not mind reading or talking about the war, but he could not bring himself to face the task of giving his parents the details he thinks they will want.'[71] As was the case in thousands of other homecomings, some things could not, and never would, be explained to friends and loved ones. 'Equally, a returned soldier's own recognition of his unique experience had the potential to make him less receptive to the well-intentioned overtures of "outsiders".'[72] Horrors were glossed over, scoffed at or effaced from individual memories, whereas the collective memory would continue to cosset the physical rather than the psychological hurt and destruction of its menfolk. 'There was a sense in which every soldier who had seen active combat and returned home thinking idealistically of his pre-war domestic life, was traumatised.[73] For some, the longed-for return home would be disillusioning. 'Yet before the last veterans reached home the cheers were already dying away, and it soon became clear that the soldiers' rewards would be less than had been promised during the war.'[74]

Endnotes

1 See *New York Times*, 10 May 1918, p. 6.

2 Springthorpe, 'War Neuroses and Civil Practice' p. 279.

3 Damousi, *Freud*, p. 35.

4 MacPherson et al., *History of the Great War*, vol. II, p. 43.

5 Ibid., pp. 8–9.

6 He had been instrumental in the introduction of Victoria's 1905 *Lunacy Act*.

7 Letter from Springthorpe, 10 August 1915 and letter from Jones, 28 August 1915. AIF 498/1/693. AWM.

8 Report on Observations of Invalid Boards by Colonel Sir Harry Maudsley, September 1918, p. 6. AWM 27 376/24.

9 'The new diagnostic categories [NYDN etc.] meant that many who were formerly classified as shell-shock cases were now not entered in the books under this category. This probably explains the levelling off in the incidence of shell-shock cases from 1916.' Garton, *The Cost of War*, p. 152.
10 Peter Warfe, 'Post Traumatic Stress and the Australian Defence Force: Lessons from peace operations in Rwanda and Lebanon', in M. Evans and A. Ryan (eds.), *The Human Face of War: Killing, Fear and Chaos in Battle*, Allen & Unwin, Sydney, 2000, p. 85.
11 Butler, *Official History*, vol. III, p. 126.
12 W. A. Turner, 'Arrangements for the Care of Cases of Nervous and Mental Shock Coming from Overseas', *Lancet*, 27 May 1916, p. 1074.
13 Damousi, *Freud in the Antipodes*, p. 35.
14 Feudtner, 'Minds the Dead have Ravished', p. 391.
15 At the time of the Armistice there were 1,000 beds available for officers and 5,000 for soldiers.
16 See M. Tyquin, *Little by Little: A Centenary History of the Royal Australian Army Medical Corps*, AMHP, Sydney, 2003.
17 Minute from Colonel A. E. Shepherd, Colonel ADMS 2nd Division (DDMS), 13 February 1918. AWM 41 [280].
18 However the following observation is worthy of note: 'It is striking that in France no new concepts were formulated which gave expression to the specific image of war.' Binneveld, *From Shell Shock to Combat Stress*', p. 88.
19 Report: 'War Neurosis', 5 October 1918 by Lieutenant-Colonel J.W. Springthorpe, Officer Commanding No. 3 AGH. AWM 11 1507/24/2.
20 Indeed they laid the basis for the treatment regimes of the next war underpinned by the principles of 'proximity, immediacy and expectation.'
21 Jones and Wessely, 'Psychiatric Battle Casualties: an Intra- and Interwar Comparison', p. 243. In 1918 the US Army would establish a special division of neurology and psychiatry within its Army Medical Corps, a unique development at the time.
22 Instructions to RMOs and MOs, 9th Australian Field Ambulance, Circular No. 115, 29 January 1917. AWM 41 [285].
23 Paul Lerner, 'Psychiatry and Casualties of War in Germany, 1914-18', *Journal of Contemporary History*, 35 (1), 2000, p. 16.
24 Binneveld, *From Shell Shock to Combat Stress*, p. 118.
25 Martin Lengwiler, 'Psychiatry beyond the Asylum: the Origins of German Military Psychiatry before Word War I' in *History of Psychiatry*, vol. 14, 2001, p. 43.
26 Lerner, 'Psychiatry and Casualties of War in Germany, 1914–18', p. 27.
27 For more on this see Mosse, 'Shell-shock as social disease', p. 106.
28 J. Bourke, *Dismembering the Male: Men's Bodies, Britain and the Great War*, Reakton, London, 1996, p. 117.
29 Mosse, 'Shell-shock as social disease', p. 106.
30 Lerner, 'Psychiatry and Casualties of War in Germany', p. 16.
31 M. D. Eder, *War Shock*, W. Heinemann, London, 1917, pp. 140–1.
32 Letter to No. 2 AGH from Major D. W. Jones (AAMC), Officer Commanding No. 4 Stationary Hospital. AWM 25 885/1-5.
33 'But the choice of a particular method depended very much on the nature of the patient's disabilities and on the length of time since the onset of shellshock.' Stone, 'Shellshock and the Psychiatrists', p. 255.
34 Butler, *Official History*, vol. III, p. 126*n*.
35 J. P. Lowson, 'The Treatment of War neuroses by Abreaction of the War Shock, *MJA*, 6 November 1926, p. 621.
36 Ibid., p. 112.
37 D. M. McWhae, 'Neuroses' in *MJA*, 2 October 1920, p. 340.
38 Letter from Lieutenant-Colonel Cecil Strangman to Major-General George Cuscaden dated 15 September 1920. A2489.20/1447. NAA (Canberra).

39 Charles Myers, 'Contributions to the Study of Shell Shock' being an Account of Certain Cases treated by Hypnosis', *Lancet*, vol. II, 8 January 1916, p. 69.

40 Lieutenant-Colonel A. M. Wilson, A/ADMS, 'Moral and Mental Disorders—Shell Shock', 2nd Australian Division Report undated (c. 1918). AWM 41/659.

41 Letter to No. 2 AGH from Major D.W. Jones (AAMC), Officer Commanding No. 4 Stationary Hospital. AWM 25 885/1-5.

42 Evans and Ryan (eds.), *The Human Face of War: Killing, Fear and Chaos in Battle*, p. 7.

43 Eder, *War Shock*, p. 142.

44 This is significant because Springthorpe had had more than a nodding acquaintance with the asylum system in Victoria since the turn of the century.

45 'Moves towards encouraging soldiers to talk about their stress, and encouraging doctors to listen psychotherapeutically, signalled an important shift in dealing with psychological problems. This cure, as with the condition itself, undermined existing understandings of military medical treatment.' Bourke, *Dismembering the Male*, p. 38.

46 J. W. Springthorpe, 'Shellshock DDMS Australian Corps', c. 1917. AWM 16 4364/48/5. John Springthorpe had a long association with this field of medicine, having written his first paper on neurosis for the 1882 *Australasian Medical Gazette*.

47 Letter from Lieutenant-Colonel J.W. Springthorpe to CO, No. 3 AAH, Dartford, 11 September 1917. AWM 41 279.

48 Memorandum dated 31 May 1918, circulated to relevant hospitals in the UK (eg No.1 AAH, Harefield) by Major-General Howse. AWM 41 [658].

49 Memorandum, 4 February 1919, 'Treatment of War Neurosis in Australia', AWM 25, 885/4.

50 Feudtner, 'Minds the Dead Have Ravished', p. 402.

51 Thomson, 'Status, Manpower and Mental Fitness', p. 154.

52 R. C. Winn, 'Psychiatry in Relation to Modern Medical Practice' in *MJA*, 6 December 1930, p. 756.

53 Thomson, 'Status, Manpower and Mental Fitness', p. 154.

54 Garton, *The Cost of War*, pp. 152–3.

55 Binneveld, *From Shell Shock to Combat Stress*, p. 88.

56 Showalter, *The Female Malady*, p. 170.

57 Ben Shepherd, *A War of Nerves: Soldiers and Psychiatrists, 1914–1994*, London, 2000, pp. 54–5.

58 Springthorpe, 'War Neuroses and Civil Practice', p. 281.

59 R. H. J. Fetherston Papers, 'Fetherston's Overseas Inspection—Report 1918', File: 12/11/3479. AWM 3 DRL 251. In Britain in 1916 most experts 'all recognised contemporaneously that the pre-morbid personality was strongly predisposed to the symptoms of shell shock.' Merskey, 'Shell-Shock', p. 255.

60 W. R. Regnell, 'The Psychoneuroses of War', *MJA*, 7 June 1919, p. 455. The figure refers to the elaborate system of percentages awarded to various injuries under war pensions regulations for calculating pensions.

61 *MJA*, 18 September 1920, p. 324.

62 This reflected civilian practice and was routine in military hospitals as well. 'Without being malingers, these men generally exaggerated their disability and, as carriers of psychic contagion were a source of danger in a ward, therefore we always endeavoured as far as possible to isolate them.' A. W. Campbell, 'Remarks on some Neuroses and Psychoses in War', *MJA*, 15 April 1916, p. 323. There had also been several unfortunate incidents fourteen years earlier on Australian troop-ships returning from the Boer War where soldiers deliberately taunted mental casualties on board to provoke a reaction.

63 Butler, *Official History*, vol. III, p. 705.

64 Letter of 4 February 1919 to Major-General Sir Neville Howse VC, DMS AIF. AWM 25 885/4.

65 Report: 'The Treatment of "Neurasthenia" in Soldiers', *MJA*, 7 December 1918, p. 481.

66 Report of Officer Commanding No. 13 AAH (Broughton Hall), 12 July 1918. This was included in a file together with a report by the Principal Medical Officer 2nd Military District, 1917, AWM 32 [62].

67 *The Times Illustrated History of the War*, vol. VII, London, 1916.

68 Summary by Colonel C. C. Manifold, DDMS Australian Corps, 1 February 1918 to A.G. Butler, p. 1. AWM 41 [659].

69 'History of cases treated at Monte Video Camp Hospital, Weymouth 1919.' AWM 25 885/4.

70 As the Melbourne *Argus* reported later: 'As the AIF ceased to exist on 1 April, all the patients became the responsibility of the Repatriation Department, and the Repatriation Commission arranged to take over the entire administration of the hospitals formerly conducted by the Defence Department in Brisbane, Adelaide, Perth and Hobart'—that is, all the smaller capital cities. 'Complete control of the military hospitals at Caulfield and Randwick will be taken over by the Repatriation Department [from Defence] on July 1.' 28 June 1921, p. 6.

71 Major A. C. Fraser, (Senior Medical Officer aboard the *Kanowna)* 'Notes on three Cases of Functional Disease of the Nervous System seen during the Voyage from England to Australia', *MJA*, 22 November 1919, p. 436.

72 Dale Blair, *Dinkum Diggers: an Australian Battalion*, Melbourne University Press, 2001, p. 181.

73 Leese, *Shell Shock*, p. 133.

74 Bill Gammage, *The Broken Years*, Penguin, Melbourne, 1975, p. 270.

Chapter Six
THE MILITARY, MEDICINE, AND THE SHELL-SHOCKED SOLDIER IN AUSTRALIA

We look now at the state of psychology in Australia during the war and contemporary schools of thought in the profession itself. From there we move to acquaint ourselves with the mental health 'establishment' in the country at that time and the relationship between the Defence Department and the newly established Repatriation Department and State Lunatic authorities. We will examine the more common treatment regimes for shell-shocked soldiers before looking at the only contemporary official inquiry to be held into the whole debate within the British Empire. There follows a discussion of the Australian Army's role and its responsibility to its members, and an exploration of some of the treatment regimes for ex-servicemen and the various 'schools of thought' that drove this treatment. This approach will enable us to make sense of how neurotic soldiers went on to assimilate into postwar society—the theme of the following chapter.

The war had thrown many mental and physical wrecks onto the shores of Australian society, but there was still controversy as to how the toll could have been reduced or its victims better treated. While not apportioning 'blame' to the army, Butler represented traditional medicine in his view that 'in the matter of strictly mental disorder, neurology and the neurologists in a measure failed the profession and the army in this crisis of 1914-1918.'[1] This was, and remains, an accurate summation. The war had also assailed the professional relationship between doctor and patient. As we have seen, the medical officer at the front took on a quasi-judicial function in his assessment of neuroses.

From the General Staff to the average civilian there lurked a suspicion that these shell-shocked men might really be malingerers (consciously or otherwise). Worse still, they could be—possibly the worst insult in the British Empire—cowards. There were implications for the revered doctor-patient association that had, for almost a century, been regarded as almost sacrosanct. 'The relationship between doctor and patient was primarily military then, not medical; consequently, the manpower needs of the war institutionalised scepticism; sickness was tainted with suspicion of cowardice, dereliction of duty and moral failure.'[2] During the war there were struggles within the medical profession not only to find a definitive cause of shell shock, but to identify who was best qualified to deal with war neuroses: the RMOs or the sometimes 'radical' schools which purported to represent modern psychiatry. There were also implications for social engineering. 'The monolithic theory of hereditary degeneration upon which Victorian psychiatry had based its social and scientific vision was significantly dented' as otherwise normal males were reduced to 'mental wrecks after a few months in the trenches.'[3] C. E.W. Bean had seen the threat early and moved deftly to disenfranchise these neurotic soldiers from his celebration of nationhood.

Before proceeding it is worthwhile to look at the differences between Australia and Britain with respect to the whole issue of shell shock. Obviously the two countries had much in common especially at various shared battle fronts and in evacuation procedures and medical nomenclature. Indeed most doctors in Australia had either trained or worked in the United Kingdom and it was British scientific literature, especially the *Lancet*, that kept the Empire's doctors informed of progress in a number of specialities. As we have seen, many Australian soldiers were treated in British military hospitals for a time. But with respect to replacing the civilian mental health infrastructure with one run by uniformed staff, the Australian experience differed from that of the United Kingdom. There, in 'all areas, there was overcrowding. This became worse in 1915, when nine of the larger asylums were transferred to the War Office as emergency military hospitals. The remaining mental hospitals became crowded with displaced patients.'[4] The much smaller numbers of AIF casualties meant that the Australian military authorities could establish small specialist hospitals in Australia, thereby not draining resources of the various state asylums.[5] This is not to say that the war did not cause problems within the mental health infrastructure here. On 11 December 1915 the medical officer at No. 13 AAH (Broughton Hall) wrote to his superiors concerning staff problems. He outlined what he thought were the prerequisites for asylum staff. These included 'good physique, experience, tact, and discretion in order to carry out their duties satisfactorily.' He complained about the gross inadequacy of the orderlies with whom he had to work, decrying them as 'mere lads, averaging about 17 years of age and possess[ing] none of the qualifications mentioned.'[6] In that month the establishment was home to thirty-two patients, including several with head wounds or who were suffering from rheumatism. In the next year it averaged sixty-two patients a month.

Apart from the military's anxiety not to encroach too far on the resources of the civil mental authorities, there were other areas in which the Australian experience differed to that of the British. For example, in his assessment of the

British Army, Peter Leese concludes that 'the parameters of wartime experience, including injury and medical treatment, were strictly limited by rank.' He argues that it was rank that 'shaped the symptoms that the soldier suffered, it affected self-perception and peer-group reactions to the disorder, and it was one of the most important elements in determining patient treatment.'[7] It has also been said of the British military that the 'drain of manpower caused by shell-shock meant that medico-military concern over mental disorder centred on containment, rather than detection.' This meant that there was then little incentive to concentrate on the exclusion of 'mental defectives' from the army.[8] But this was not the Australian experience.

Rank had far less influence in Australian military medicine and indeed within the AIF itself where soldiers particularly recognised, and deferred to, ability before hierarchy and they frequently showed their displeasure if the two did not go hand-in-hand. Both in Australia and abroad senior officers of the AAMC constantly fought against government demands to relax recruiting standards. This is not to say that thousands did not slip through the net in 1914 and 1915. But thereafter the system was tightened with due regard to identifying recruits with potential mental problems. But selection was still more an art than a science. Of *all* the 589,947 recruits to the AIF who were examined during the First World War, fewer than 178,800 were rejected on medical grounds with the tightening of screening procedures as the war progressed. Of these 178,800, only a very small number (1.44%) were rejected for 'Disorders of the Mind', but on the same grounds a further 4.86% recruits were subsequently identified in training camps around Australia.[9] Like those rejected initially on physical grounds, the number of recruits actually identified with psychological problems is probably an under-representation.

The Mental Health Establishment in Australia

Each state in Australia (which only federated in 1901) possessed its own infrastructure and legislation to deal with mental defectives and the administration of asylums. Not unnaturally much of this legal and organisational structure was modelled on that of Great Britain, with the important exception that there was not the encumbrance of its Poor Law legislation. However the antipodean infrastructure was minuscule by comparison and the larger states (on the basis of population) had to take the lead. In 1901 the head of the Victorian Lunacy Service had called for the establishment of early treatment facilities in general hospitals. Then, in 1914, the 'amendment of the lunacy legislation enabled voluntary patients to be legally admitted to state hospitals for the insane, receiving houses and private licensed establishments.'[10] This provided little stimulation, however, within the medical profession itself. As A. G. Butler admitted, in Australian medical schools 'the teaching of neurology and psychiatry was in line with that elsewhere; neither had much concern with the "mental" and "psychological" attributions of their speciality.'[11] The war did spur some legislative amendments, however. For example, on 3 November 1915 the Victorian Government gazetted its *Mental Treatment Act (1915)* specifically to enable its institutions to care for ex-military personnel for up to six months. Certainly across the Tasman in New Zealand the starting point of modern psychiatry there has been identified as the First World War.[12]

At the time of the outbreak of war there were no trained analysts practising in Australia, nor were there any specialist clinics or psychoanalytic institutes as existed in Britain and on the continent. Because Freud's ideas and practices were adopted in 'a selective and eclectic way' some mainstream physicians 'were resistant to interpretations of the role of sexuality', especially homosexuality, in repression and trauma. Put simply, they 'lacked the specialised knowledge to understand its importance.'[13] There were very few practitioners in Australia in 1915 who could lay claim to having mastered Freudian techniques. 'The physician's attitude toward the hysteric and the neurasthenic was often one of moral condemnation: they were seen as morally depraved, wilful and egoistic.'[14] This view is most evident in reading Butler's medical history of the war and it was an attitude shared both by his mentor C. E.W. Bean and the senior Australian military hierarchy.

Australian society, like most others in the West, regarded mental illness—'insanity'—with a mixture of fascination and dread: fascination because of the bizarre ways patients sometimes presented with their symptoms and dread arising from their own self-doubt. There was then a stigma attached to those suffering with neurosis. Returned soldiers and their relatives were acutely aware of this and did not want to add to what many of them already saw as their private shame. They teetered on the edge of a society whose moral keepers were fickle in their assessment of who was fit to belong. 'Shell-shock was a legal, medical and moral half-way house in a society used to a clear division between the mad and the sane.'[15] Returned soldiers' groups and regimental associations were highly sensitive to the problem and lobbied to ensure there would be no such stain on their colleagues' reputation as returned soldiers. Most of their efforts went to ensure that their mates were not 'certified'—the final shame for anyone entering the mental health system of the time. To be certified meant one had abrogated one's rights and responsibilities. The stigma of certification had been earlier recognised in the civilian sphere and was well understood by the wider public. Speaking in 1911, South Australia's Chief Asylum Officer, Dr M. Downey, noted that 'the certification of insanity often entails undeserved hardship on the person who after recovery from an attack seeks to resume his place in the social world.'[16]

But the issue of certification also posed problems for the states, which were genuinely sympathetic and eager to help men and women from the services. Indeed the problem vexed a number of government departments both at the commonwealth and state level. On 15 October 1917 the Secretary of the Defence Department wrote to his equivalent in the Repatriation Department concerning the admission of soldiers to civilian asylums in the various military districts around Australia and highlighting the complications of the current system. 'Unfortunately the State laws in almost all districts do not allow mental cases to be treated in mental asylums unless they are certified as lunatics. This is the case in Queensland, South Australia and Tasmania. In Victoria a special Act was passed that all soldiers might be treated in Mental Asylums without certification, and in New South Wales while no Act was passed, this was possible under the existing Act.'[17]

Despite political goodwill and the appropriate physical resources and staffing levels characteristic of the state systems, soldiers were still loath to leave ad hoc military mental hospitals (as they were early in the war) to enter the civilian system, even though the Commonwealth had guaranteed that they would not be certified on admission. At an important conference of medical military officers in Melbourne in 1918 one officer indicated just how deeply this fear was held. He reported that there should not be any link or association between 'neurasthenic patients' and mental cases, as the implied connection was a nightmare for the former. He then recalled a patient at No. 5 AGH whom, when told he would be sent to No. 16 (Mont Park Mental Hospital) had an immediate relapse. He maintained that 'if an institution is established for neurasthenic patients it should be a separate institution, kept only for such patients.'[18]

In some cases this anxiety was magnified by the press as illustrated in this editorial from the *Argus* from 11 July 1921. The issue concerned ninety-seven men in the Mont Park Military Hospital who were suffering as a result of their wartime experiences. The State Lunacy Department had applied for them to be transferred to civilian asylums. Strong feelings had been aroused and subsequent public discussion indicated that 'the treatment now being received by the soldiers and that given to civilian patients is different, and release from the civil institutions is more difficult.'[19] As least once in 1921 the Minister for Repatriation had personally intervened at the eleventh hour to prevent a soldier being transferred from a military facility, in this case No. 16 AGH, to a civilian asylum. The Returned Sailors and Soldiers Imperial League of Australia (Victoria), the Soldier's Mothers'

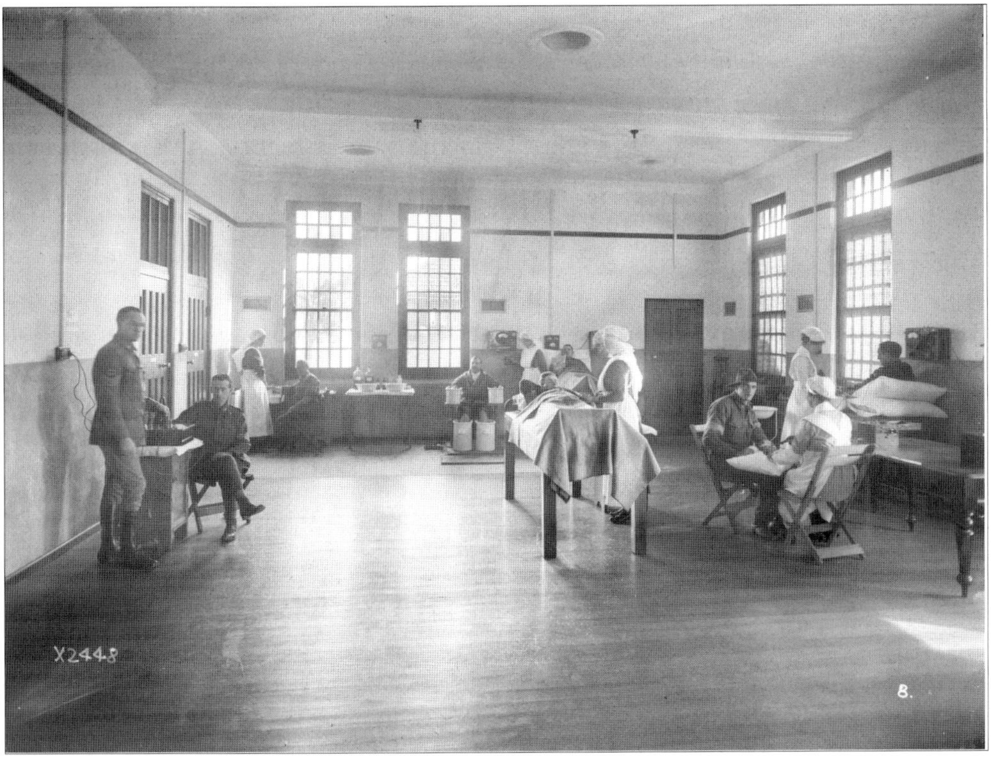

A ward scene at Victoria's Mont Park Hospital c. 1919.
Some of these electrical appliances were used in an attempt to alleviate
the symptoms of shell-shocked patients.
(AWM DAX248)

Association, various other women's groups, and the Fathers' Association of the R.S.S.I.L.A. were vocal critics of such attempts to place soldiers in mainstream mental health care. Their compassion was often misplaced however, because these were usually the very places best able to help these men.[20]

With respect to those civilian asylums identified as being suitable for treating military members, arrangements came at a cost and threw up questions of power. Victoria's Inspector General of the Insane wrote to the Minister of Defence in 1917: 'It is necessary, taking into consideration the mental condition of these patients, that they should be in charge of men holding some military rank—otherwise difficulties will arise in the minds of military patients receiving instructions from an attendant who is either a civilian or ranks merely as a private.'[21] The question of finance was determined variously between the states. In Victoria, for example, financial arrangements had been made as early as 1915 which determined that 'the cost of mental patients was between £13/21/2 to £29/41/2 [shillings] per week per patient.' A later addition to this arrangement saw the Commonwealth undertake to pay Victoria one pound per week for the care and attendance of critical patients. The Commonwealth would also pay thirty shillings for patients who did not actually reside in Victoria, 'the reason being that the State authorities desired that they themselves should bear some of the expense for Victorian patients...[although they did not think] it right, that they should bear the expense of cases from other States.'[22]

In South Australia, however, the Repatriation Department took up an offer by a qualified nursing sister in the private sector to receive military patients at her Erindale Rest Home, Burnside, at a rate of £2/2/- per week, which she pointed out 'is below the minimum fee for private patients.'[23] She was also given the honorary rank of sister in the Australian Army Nursing Service—after all, discipline had to be maintained in the wards. In Western Australia, No. 24 AAH had been established at 'Stromness' in Cottesloe and its officer commanding was Captain J. T. Anderson, a part-time officer who was also Inspector General for the Insane in that state. Professional asylum doctors who were given part-time commissions in the army almost always held such appointments. 'Stromness' opened on 4 March 1918 and was 'a very suitable building with grounds ample for recreation and a vegetable garden for instruction of patients.' Market gardens and domestic animals such as milk cows and poultry were important ways through which these modest establishments could keep costs down. By July 1918 it had thirteen patients and a staff of seven non-commissioned officers and soldiers. Forty-nine patients had been admitted during the year, two had died, and thirty ex-soldiers had been discharged.[24]

During the war, when a number of war neuroses patients were either still being treated in England or were en route home, the numbers being cared for around Australia were still relatively small. The figures published for Victoria in 1917 are not untypical.[25] The interesting feature here is the incidence of soldiers who had never left Australia.

'Soldiers Treated in "Hospitals for the Insane" by the Victorian Lunacy Department since the beginning of the war until 31 July 1917.'

"Overseas Men":

RECEIVED	DISCHARGED	DIED	REMAINING RESIDENT	REMAINING ON TRIAL
10	6	-	2	2

"Prior To Embarkation Men" (never left Australia):

RECEIVED	DISCHARGED	DIED	REMAINING RESIDENT	REMAINING ON TRIAL
76	6	4	-	8

New South Wales, with the largest population and the biggest concentration of medical professionals, also managed to cope despite the rising numbers of in-patients. 'During the year ending 30 June 1918, the total number of cases of nerve strain, including shell shock, neurasthenia and cases with pronounced mental symptoms, admitted has been 333 which is an increase of 196 over the corresponding period of the previous year's report.' From the time Broughton Hall in Sydney was opened on 21 October 1915, to the end of 1918, it had admitted 574 cases. According to its superintendent, the 'mental disturbance' of most of his soldier patients was 'transitory', ending in complete recovery, although such optimism was not always well founded. He was quite candid in adding that 'suitable accommodation is provided for cases for which the mental symptoms are more marked.'[26]

Contemporary Psychological Schools of Thought

Away from the front, war neuroses were generally managed by one or a combination of simplified 'psychotherapeutic treatment'. These were persuasion, explanation, suggestion, analysis, re-education and occupation. The fact that the empire was at war with the home of Freudian and other sophisticated Austro-German schools of psychology did not help matters. After all, if Beethoven were now proscribed, there was little hope of airing Germanic psychiatric theories. Despite popular opposition from many medical quarters 'Freudian theory provided the only real language to explain hysteria. Even among doctors (notably A. G. Butler), who found the doctrines of Freud preposterous the arguments that hysteria represented an "unconscious flight into illness"...gained their particular impetus from the Viennese analyst.'[27] During the war various military hospitals became recognised focal points for the varying theories on how best to deal with shell-shocked soldiers. Some continued after the war, but the practitioners who worked at these places moved to private practice, clinics or, in rare cases, public hospitals, to continue their work.

The major British centres included Craiglockhart, Maghull, Netley, Golders Green, and Napsbury, and were usually established on, or worked along lines of, rigid rank hierarchy.[28] The AIF either sent its own casualties to these places or accommodated them in small auxiliary hospitals scattered about the British countryside such as at Seale Hayne and Dartford. Doctors as varied as their psychological regimes staffed these institutions. They included British anthropologist W. H. R. Rivers, Charles Myers, R.G. Rows, L. R. Yealland (an 'enthusiastic' Canadian), and Ernest Jones (not to be confused with an Australian doctor of the same name at the same period). In Australia, C. G. Godfrey, A. T. Edwards, W. R. Regnell, J. P. Lowson, and Ernest Jones were the leading proponents of psychology. But even some of these continued to labour under the pervasive influence of the concept of inheritance in insanity.[29] Not everyone was happy with the British system, however, and one Australian doctor believed that mental cases 'of long standing' were the result 'of wrong diagnosis and wrong treatment and most special neurological hospitals in England are museums of medical failure.'[30]

These 'streams' within the discipline of psychology may be further distilled into three main schools of thought. One large group of doctors, including some military doctors and British Ministry of Pensions officials (often effectively the same thing) focused on physical shock, concussion, and hereditary causes. 'When they failed to explain a case they argued for some form of moral degeneracy.' Both C.E.W. Bean and A. G. Butler belong to this category. 'There were also two schools of psychological explanation: a smaller group influenced by psychoanalytic ideas, and a group with a more widespread pragmatic approach that contained both progressive and disciplinary wings.'[31] Even hypnosis with its 'savour of the uncanny, the mysterious and the unknown' was frowned upon by the military in both Britain and Australia. In Britain, the army's senior psychologist, Lieutenant-Colonel Charles Myers, caused a stir with his methods. He was told by the commandant of one military hospital 'that he would in no circumstances countenance its employment because the reputation of his unit would suffer thereby.'[32]

L. R. Yealland and W. H. R. Rivers have been described as representing 'the two poles of psychiatric modernism.'[33] These two doctors' approach to shell shock illustrates some of the critical differences in methods of curing the shell-shocked soldier. What did they stand for and in what ways were their methods different? The Canadian Lewis Yealland, a deft hand at applying electric shocks to his patients, represented 'the quick fix' and stood for discipline within British psychology (and in this he shared something with his German contemporaries) and clearly thought that shell shock was really hysteria in khaki. His forte was 'faradic' treatment, or the application of repeated electric shocks to his patients. There was little sympathy for the subject in these sadistic practices. He noted:

> The treatment is best carried out in a special room set apart for the purpose, where there will be nothing to distract the patients attention...The patient is given no time to collect his thoughts, but is hurried along by a mixture of persuasion and command until the disordered function has completely recovered. The patient is never allowed any say in the matter...Rapidity and an authoritative manner are the chief factors in the re-education process.'[34]

It seems that most of his patients 'came from the ranks, and his blatant use of power and authority was part of the therapy.'[35] There was also an arrogance in his rationale, to wit: 'The therapeutic uses of electricity are still mysterious enough to the layman, and nearly every patient is willing to accept the suggestion that some form of electricity will cure him.'[36] At the time, some Australian psychologists were appalled and Paul Dane was to write a scathing view of this practice in 1950. 'To treat a traumatic neurosis by shock methods is entirely unjustifiable and betrays an ignorance of psychopathology so profound that a doctor in a civil practice would be ruined.'[37]

Nor did Yealland listen to his patients, for whom he seemed to have a poor regard. 'The chief phenomena underlying the hysterical type of mind are weakness of the will and of the intellect, hyper-suggestibility and negativism. The majority of patients are below the average scale of intelligence...and others who are more highly equipped prove to have an unstable history either personally or in the family.'[38] Yealland was one of many 'disciplinary therapists' who 'collapsed any distinction between legitimate neurosis and malingering.' His task was to make 'the consequences of the symptom painful and to persuade the patient to relinquish it and resume his official, soldierly and manly function.'[39] Although he claimed a ninety-five per cent success rate in curing mutism, deafness, paraplegia etc, for all his efforts he did not move past 'hysteria' as the only legitimate term to describe what he was dealing with in military hospitals on a daily basis.

But if the soldier's unconscious desire to cheat the army of his share of labour had to be excised, his deeper subconscious remained untouched by the non-Freudians. Their reluctance to fully understand Freud's theories limited what treatments could be used as well as their efficacy. Even before the war the medical establishment had deplored Freud's originality as 'perverted'. Subsequently this body did not move much from its predominantly moral stand until after the Second World War.

Even among Freud's disciples in Britain, this aspect of his approach to psychology went against Edwardian prudery. Dr W. Rivers adopted Freud's views on psychoanalysis but, unlike other advocates of Freudian techniques (for example the neurologist Ernest Jones), he baulked at the one 'that most offended pragmatic British medical sensibilities...Where he departed from Freud was in the function of sexual aetiology in neurosis.'[40] Like Myers, Butler, Springthorpe and others he claimed that sex had little to do with shell shock. 'Rather than tracing the origins of the hysterical and anxiety states associated with shellshock back to the patient's infantile sexual impulses, Rivers centred his aetiological account on the emotional world of the battlefield.'[41] The employment of psychoanalytic techniques by some members of both the RAMC and the AAMC always proceeded in the face of 'entrenched psychiatric opposition'. What success it did enjoy was due to the fact that those 'military doctors who used Freudian insights to treat distraught servicemen largely ignored the sexual foundations of the therapeutic program.'[42]

Others who professed to share common ground with Freud 'however much we may disapprove or be *disgusted* [emphasis added] with the methods and theories of the psycho-analytical school', were not comfortable with this aspect of the Austrian's work. Melbourne doctor W. R. Regnell firmly believed that the treatment by psycho-therapy should not be carried out along Freudian lines. His view was that war neuroses proved 'the universal sex theory of causation of the neuroses was no longer tenable, we must allow that in the treatment of the neuroses we owe much to the researches of Freud.'[43] He was also probably ahead of his time which was, ironically, an unfortunate outcome for neurotic soldiers for, although 'arguments about shell shock helped establish the Freudian notion that hysterical symptoms were due to emotional conflict, they also undermined the relationship that Freud alleged between these symptoms and childhood sexual experiences.'[44]

The medical superintendent of Melbourne's Kew Mental Hospital also 'condemned psychoanalysis as the outpouring of the "morbid minded, one might say, paratypical sexual occultist of Vienna".' Such disdain continued into the twenties and thirties as leading psychiatrists 'dismissed the theory as "balderdash" and its practitioners as "charlatans".'[45] But eventually it was shell shock which weighted the medical profession's views 'in favour of Freud's theory of emotional conflict in hysteria, but against the notion of an infantile sexual aetiology.'[46] The otherwise enlightened J.W. Springthorpe penned his view of psychoanalysis in the *Medical Journal of Australia*, suggesting that was it was no exaggeration to say that 'war neuroses have completely shattered the original perverted notion of a sexual basis and driven such Freudism to oblivion.'[47]

Morally conservative views among most members of Australia's medical profession inevitably hindered the effective and timely management of hundreds of shell-shocked soldiers for the next decade or so. It also retarded individual careers including, for example, a former AAMC officer and later eminent psychologist, Paul Dane. It has been argued that Dane's belief 'in the strict application of psychoanalytic practice following Freud's prescription put him in a minority, especially in his views on the centrality of sexuality.'[48]

Views such as his would also have been anathema to C.E.W. Bean and A. G. Butler. During the twenties Dane worked with neurotic soldiers through the application of 'Freudian and psychoanalytic methods'. He argued that their problems stemmed from repressing sexual desire. He also revealed the frequency

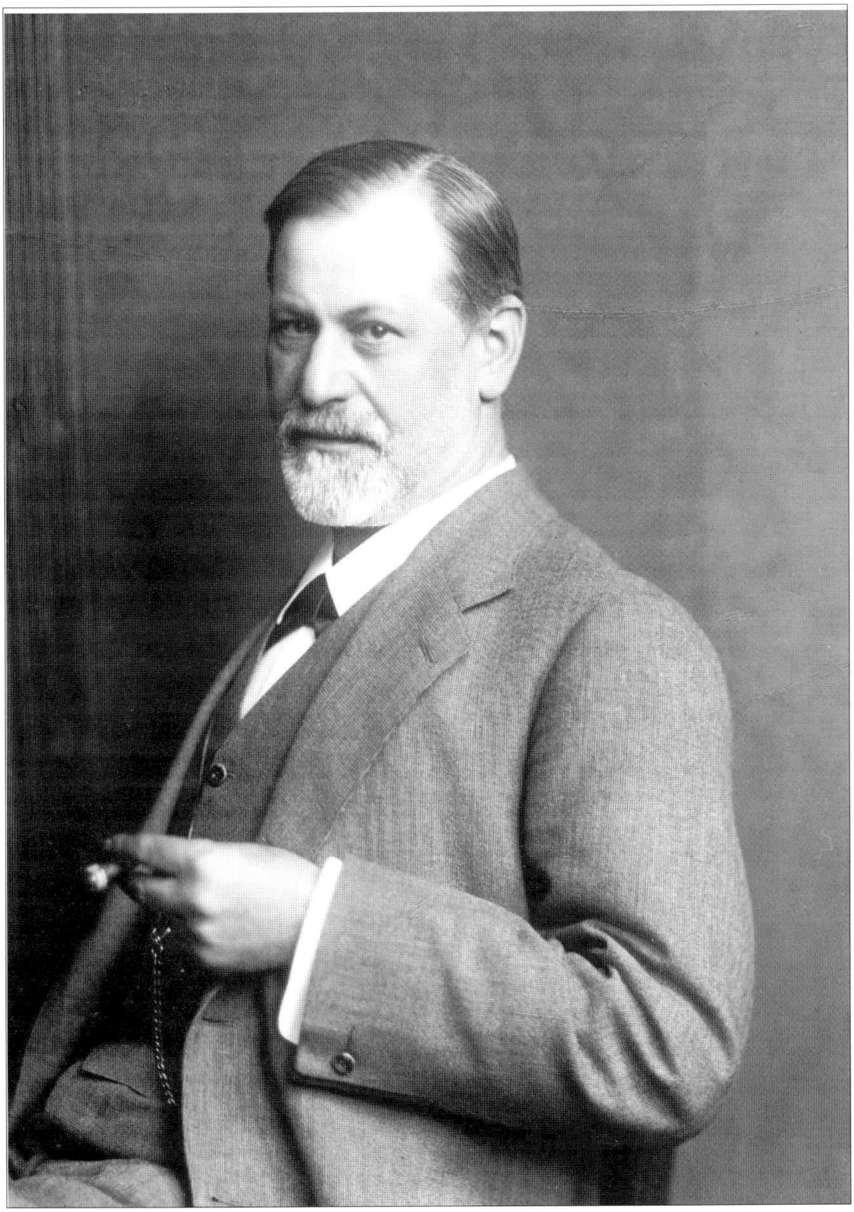

Sigmund Freud. The Austrian psychologist provided a glimmer of light in the early years of military psychiatry. Even he underestimated the longevity of neuroses such as shell shock.

with which these men 'will tell of sexual abnormality.'[49] Dane was not afraid to nail his colours to the mast of psychology and wrote that, while he believed many British psychologists accepted parts of 'Freudian mechanism', they tended to believe that symptoms of war neurosis were brought on by fear. But for Dane 'the problems of the pyscho-neurosis can be understood only on the lines laid down by Freud.'[50] Apart from individuals, institutions could also make their mark on the psychology debate. The War Office and other army authorities stood to lose face if the shell shock epidemic was explained away in terms that left them in a bad light and which might have unknown consequences for another war. In Britain it was decided to exorcise this slur on military honour by establishing an inquiry.

The 1922 Committee of Inquiry into Shell Shock

The special investigation into shell shock arose from a debate in the House of Lords on 28 April 1920. As a consequence the War Office (hardly an impartial player) appointed a committee 'to consider the different types of hysteria and traumatic neuroses commonly called shell shock...' The committee sat from 7 September 1920 to 22 June 1922 and, over forty-one sittings, heard fifty-nine witnesses. Its findings were published in August 1922 (coincidentally, at the same time, the British official medical history of the war was about to go to print). The committee attached great importance 'to the effect of discipline, moral, esprit de corps, training, leadership, selection of *suitable* [emphasis added] regimental officers, and rest and comfort in the prevention of nervous disorders on active service.'[51] It was clear that the committee would support the War Office view that it was the soldier, not the war, which was to blame for his mental state. It was significant that the British Army's own senior consultant psychologist, Colonel C. S. Myers, had quit in 1917 'in a state of utter disillusionment with the medical authorities and he subsequently refused to give evidence' before the committee.[52] Most of the witnesses (few of whom served at the front during any of the major battles) appeared to share common prejudices. They believed that the stress of war *rarely* produced insanity in the relatively stable man. But war would have acted "as is commonly observed with other forms of stress' on men who 'by predisposition were liable to breakdown.'[53]

Prewar somatic theories of the origins of mental illness were intermittently reasserted by the committee, and Freud and his 'sexual' theories were 'explicitly rejected.'[54] From the evidence placed before it, the committee concluded that at least eighty per cent of combined British and French cases were purely emotional, while only five per cent could be attributed to concussion. Even after the war, medicine took a back seat to morality and willpower, those keystones of empire. The 1922 inquiry 'rejected even the most modified forms of psychiatric treatment, and both medical and military authorities treating war neurotic ex-servicemen held the same opinion.'[55] Some see this inquiry as an attempt by the British military establishment 'to distance itself from the psychiatric spillage of the war, to minimise its cultural significance, and to reinstate in the public mind a more traditional moral vision.'[56] Australia dutifully toed the line abetted by the official histories (of C.E.W. Bean and A. G. Butler), that were then about to come into general circulation. The War Office Committee's conclusion defiantly reasserted prewar military values, as if the shell shock crisis had altered nothing.

Treatment in Australia

Doctor W. E. Jones was Inspector General of the Insane in Victoria and for a time had been superintendent of the Radnor Asylum in Wales. He wrote that, from his perspective, the 'most interesting class of cases we are beginning to see, inasmuch as they are most difficult of explanation, are those in which grave temporary disturbance of the special senses occurs.'[57] His paper, submitted to the *Medical Journal of Australia*, also reflected the confusion among specialists in the United Kingdom as he noted what new, and seemingly contradictory, clinical British publications had to say.

One modern scholar has described this aspect of rehabilitation eloquently. While military physicians 'strove to return men to active service, they targeted their therapy at different aspects of the incapacitation and employed a wide range of techniques.'[58] One of the basic differences in approach concerned the mechanism of psychological injury—in other words, how had the casualty arrived at this mental state? As we have seen, some understood shell shock as 'organic'—a physical or neurological condition with as yet undiscovered microscopic lesions causing soldiers to lose their mental balance. Others took a more sophisticated view and held that the problem was indeed a psychiatric one. As in Britain, psychological care in Australia ran the full gamut from poorly understood sessions of hypnosis to electric shock. During and after the war, medicine and psychology generally took the lead from developments and trends in Britain and the United States. Here, the two major streams incorporated the 'moral view of neurosis that fashioned disciplinary treatments' which contrasted sharply with 'the "analytic" view, which is best represented by, but by no means identical with, psycho-analysis.'[59]

So there formed a divide between those who supported or practised some form of Freudian therapy, and those, especially in military circles, who believed Freud was too obsessed with sex and infantile impulses to be taken seriously. Despite acknowledging Freud as 'legitimate' and a leader in the field of psychiatry, A. G. Butler's attitude was typical of most, but by no means all, of his AAMC colleagues.[60] While damning many of his theories, Freud's opponents still selected those parts of his terminology that suited their own views or prejudices. Whatever one's leanings, the influx of shell-shocked casualties meant that Australian 'psychiatry was faced with unprecedented challenges during World War I when the effective treatment of war neuroses demanded psycho-dynamic approaches which were at odds with the prevailing organic conceptions of psychiatry.'[61] Both the military and the medical establishment in Australia had been caught flat-footed in the face of this epidemic of 'madness'. The public was as confused as were the afflicted. As the war creaked along, the army belatedly realised that the individual was not to blame for neurotic episodes such as shell shock and this forced the authorities to look for psychological explanations. It was a small victory for its psychiatric casualties.

Despite the lack of unity in managing neurotic soldiers, the army, in contrast to its earlier recruiting procedures, generally evolved an efficient system for getting these men into appropriate centres for treatment. As early as 1917 all patients returning from the front and destined for the eastern seaboard were landed by ship in Melbourne (then the federal capital) and placed in military hospitals there. After clinical observation and further scrutiny by medical staff, they were returned to the military district responsible for them. Local military authorities then found these soldiers suitable accommodation and placed them under the care of psychologists drawn from that state's lunatic services while the Defence Department (and later the Repatriation Commission) paid for their treatment and board. Both the Inspectors General for the Insane in New South Wales and Victoria were given army commissions in the AAMC to facilitate the efficient management of this process.[62] By June 1918 the following military hospitals for mental patients existed around the country: Broughton Hall, New South Wales (71 beds); Mont Park, Victoria (42 beds); and Cottesloe, Western Australia (30 beds).[63] Men from the less populated states were routinely sent to one of these facilities.

Since 1917 the policy of the Defence Department had been that no soldier whose mental trouble had been caused by active service outside Australia should be certified as a lunatic until it could be proved that his case was either incurable or extremely chronic. Soldiers whose mental problems had been detected prior to their embarking overseas were discharged in monthly drafts and handed over

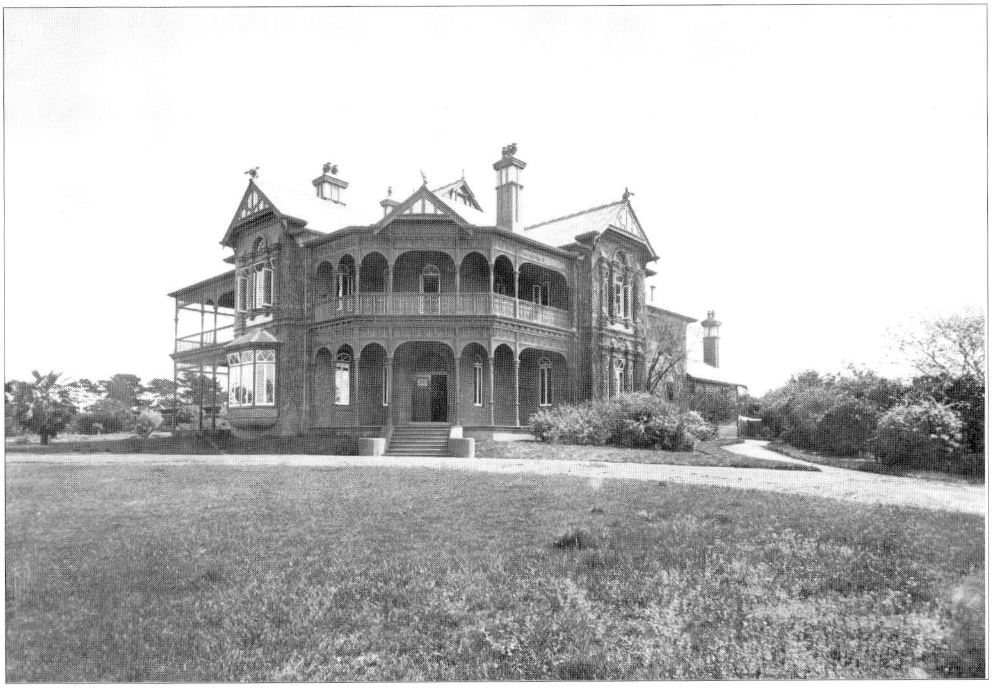

Not a film set for a Hitchcock thriller, the imposing photograph of one of the army's special hospitals (Bundoora, c.1920) for the shell-shocked belied the careful and sympathetic treatment these casualties received on their return from Europe.
(AWM H12896)

to the various state lunatic authorities. In other words they were not treated 'in the same manner as those men whose mental trouble has been caused through stress of active service.' This was done in a separate 'stream.' Where appropriate these men were given over to the care of their family or parents 'if the military authorities are satisfied that this can be done and the applicants are proper persons to have charge of them, *violent men excluded*.'[64] The latter were usually placed under restraint in the only places that had the appropriate facilities—civilian asylums.

All parties were keen to stress to ex-service patients, to their families, and to the general public, that there was no shame in being admitted to one of these establishments. As Colonel Eric Sinclair, a leading Australian psychiatrist, wrote to Major-General Richard Fetherston, the senior military medical officer in Australia: 'Residence in such an institution does not, of itself, indicate that the patient suffered from mental disease, and, being a military hospital, admission is obtained by the usual transfer without certificate of any kind...' Here was a tacit admission on the part of the military medical authorities that such mental problems did, in fact, stem from the casualties' active service. We now see the beginnings of a divergence from official British attitudes in the same period. Sinclair had also attended the June 1918 conference in Melbourne and he represented a growing opinion in not wanting to see any ex-soldier 'being discharged before cure, rather than the usual procedure during the war, of discharging them after six months.'[65] All the other medical officers present shared this view—but not everyone there was convinced that all sufferers were what they seemed. Elsewhere other Australian medical officers persisted with the malingerer theory. Two years later Lieutenant-Colonel Cecil Strangman could still write to General George Cuscaden, the new Director General of Medical Services, stating that, in treating neuropathic men 'disciplinary measures may be necessary when dealing with a few of them.'[66]

The Australian Army's senior consultant psychologist, Colonel Sir Harry Maudsley, reported on the proceedings of a number of invalid boards towards the end of the war. 'Most of these cases of war neuroses were of good physique and judging from their previous history, were of good "mental makeup", but there were many of poorish physique and with histories pointing to a poor mental makeup. Men ready to suffer from neurosis on the slightest provocation. Some failed to complete their training and a considerable number had not been at the front.'[67] The time-honoured 'school' of suspicion and mistrust of the shell-shocked soldier was a resilient one and it still had adherents in high places.

Elsewhere, screening procedures were tightened in an effort to reduce the number of actual or potential psychiatric cases who joined the services. Private X of the 9th Battalion had enlisted in the army early in May 1915, despite an instance of mental breakdown twelve months previously which included a four-month stay in a mental hospital. Repatriated to Australia (hence the government's concern at the drain on public finances, not to mention the drain on the AAMC's resources) he was admitted to Broughton Hall with 'mania'. This soldier had managed to serve in Egypt for nine months without any apparent difficulty, but while in France he was in no fewer than six military hospitals during 1917 suffering from 'depression' and 'delusion'.[68] His was not an isolated case. Reference has already been made to the poor screening of recruits in Australia in 1914 and 1915. The professional literature in Australia and the popular press now began to confirm earlier realisations by the AAMC of the long-term implications of poor recruit screening. 'The possibility of a person of marked mental deficiency enlisting for active service with the Australian Imperial Force has been demonstrated in a case which engaged the attention of the Criminal Court, Perth...It appears that the man in question had been recognised to be mentally deficient during the whole of his life.'[69] The soldier in question had enlisted in 1915 but he was not discharged until March 1918, having in the interim being promoted to lance-corporal. He was later charged with having committed a sexual offence and was released into the care of an asylum.

Twenty-two-year-old Sergeant W, 19th Battalion, had, in the one incident, been gassed and then hurled into the air by the force of an artillery shell, while at Pozières in September 1916. He was unconscious at the start of what was becoming a typical odyssey for shell-shocked victims. He was evacuated to Etaples where he spent a fortnight before being transferred to the 2nd Eastern General Hospital, Brighton, for two weeks. From there he was admitted to Dartford for four days then sent to No.1 Command Depot for a month. There the sergeant was finally discharged (after undergoing who knows what forms of treatment) from hospital, but kept on duty. Back in Australia in October 1918, he was diagnosed with neurasthenia and reportedly 'has been getting thinner and more nervous.'[70] What made it more difficult for treating doctors in Australia after 1918 was the loss of comprehensive medical records (see Appendix One). If the patient's memory was not good and typically with neurotic soldiers this was usually the case, medical staff had some difficulty trying to retrace the steps of others who had treated their patients in the early stages of their condition.

Once the Armistice was signed in 1918 moves began to set matters on a firmer footing than had been possible during the war. Across the country more permanent arrangements were made for the continuing treatment of ex-servicemen. In Victoria No. 14 AAH at Macleod closed on 26 March 1918 and its patients were transferred to the newly opened No.16 AGH. Purpose-built by the state government as a 178-bed hospital for the insane, it was handed over to the Defence Department and assumed a distinctly military atmosphere. A staff sergeant-major led the physically fit in daily exercises for patients with heart, lung and neurasthenic conditions on the lines laid down by the Hampstead Hospital in Britain during the war. As many as sixty to seventy men participated daily and, according to Dr John Springthorpe, the results were 'very gratifying'. But what continued to upset him after his return from the war was the tardiness with which some elements of the repatriation system were adopting and implementing new overseas research and practices and adapting these to suit local conditions. Referring to neurological cases, he wrote that he had had found that local medical boards, whose members usually had no experience at the front, had simply discharged many ex-servicemen 'as malingerers and without any pension.' This error was compounded further by the men being 'quite wrongly treated with isolation and restraint.'[71] Springthorpe had previously been elected by the Pensions Department as Commonwealth

Medical Referee for neurological cases and retained his keen interest in their welfare after the war.

Treatment of the shell-shocked or neurotic soldier at public expense was predicated on his condition's being caused by a physical or psychological injury. A soldier's subsequent management and treatment followed from this, even though the diagnosis of his problem might change over time and in different institutions or even under different doctors. Many followers of both approaches, however, still laboured under the nineteenth century constructs of hereditary predisposition that would continue to distract them until the late 1930s.[72] There were dissenters, however, even early in the war. In a departure from the view generally held by both medicine and the military, M. D. Eder proposed that 'war-shock is hysteria occurring in a person free from hereditary or personal psycho-neurotic antecedents, but with a mind more responsive to psychical stimulus than the normal.'[73] But practitioners seemed to forget that, in not screening out mental defectives, the army's own recruiting process had effectively failed.

The Army's Responsibilities

As we have seen, army authorities were reluctant to discharge mentally wounded men until they believed them to have been completely 'cured.' Two main reasons for retaining men in the service until this outcome was achieved have been suggested: 'The first was to ensure that soldiers would not contaminate society after demobilisation. The second was to reduce the likelihood of a pension being granted on psychiatric grounds in civil life.'[74] This was, after all, a time when the insane were incarcerated and isolated from the wider community and perhaps this reflected unspoken public anxieties. Too much can be made of individuals such as A. G. Butler's personal fears linked to his interest in eugenics that accompanied a natural scepticism. The second argument concerning pensions is an over-generalisation and cannot be sustained on the extant documentary evidence, despite the well-articulated, and therefore most widely disseminated, views of some senior army officers, public servants and politicians.

Many commanders, field officers and army medical men genuinely believed that the army owed its psychiatric and other mental casualties the best care possible in the hope of a cure, prior to demobilisation. At one stage a policy existed which determined that no-one suffering from mental illness could be discharged within six months of returning to Australia. However not everyone was happy with this approach. One army officer stated his misgivings at the 17

June 1918 conference previously mentioned. This meeting had been organised specifically to discuss the mental health of returning soldiers and the issue of how best to care for them. Major S. Sewel was one of those who opposed the six month policy. He was a member of one of the repatriation boards and explained that he was seeing men who, even after three years of treatment, were 'almost as bad as when they were discharged.' These ex-soldiers returned to civilian life after being demobilised and had tried various jobs and trades without success. Sewel explained that they had now become 'a burden on the State' and he thought this was the army's fault. He argued for a period longer than six months. 'They should be allowed to join work classes and be got physically fit before they are discharged.' Some war neurotics had even come back to him and asked to be returned to hospital and he predicted that 'there are hundreds of men who are apparently going to be quite useless for the rest of their lives unless some action is going to be taken to hold them.'[75]

He appears to have argued his case successfully. In reporting this meeting, the *Medical Journal of Australia* stated that psychological casualties would now 'be retained under the control of the military authorities for such period of time as was considered necessary...epileptic soldiers and the incurable inebriates should be retained by the military authorities for the purpose of medical treatment, and that these patients might be referred to the Department of Repatriation.'[76]

Britain, Canada and the United States paid pensions on the grounds of mental illness. Until the massive burden of war reparations ruined Germany's economy, she had done the same. But France was different. It was with perhaps grudging admiration that Britain's official medical historian of the war wrote that the 'point-blank refusal of the French authorities to admit the legitimacy of non-organic war injury meant that they avoided the dilemmas that dogged the British Army.' With no term like 'shell shock' to imply physical damage, 'all neurotics were by definition malingerers. Moreover, as there was no organic condition to register or measure, and no discharge from the French Army without admission of full cure, the question of a pension never arose.'[77] The difference could not have been starker. Apart from the critical importance of an income to the individual ex-soldier and his family or dependants, pensions have subsequently been used as a statistical tool to gauge the extent of mental illness among the Australian population of returned servicemen. The number of pensions allocated to returned World War I soldiers suggests that there was a significant problem. 'By 1930 there were 12,844 veterans receiving pensions on psychiatric grounds and, by 1939, 4,891 cases of war neurosis had been treated in repatriation facilities. In this case, war neurosis included shell shock, epilepsy, neurasthenia and alcoholism.'[78]

While some writers have seen this as a mean-spirited approach by officialdom to pensions during and immediately after the war, there is little evidence to suggest that a similar approach was adopted in the mental health sphere. In some ways this argues the success of contemporary perceptions by servicemen's associations and advocates of perceived injustices in the system. The uncritical acceptance of these highly successful marketing ploys has continued with little reassessment ever since. Letters such as this one from the Officer Commanding No. 13 AAH setting out contemporary standard procedures are typical. 'As soon as incapacity can be estimated by the [Medical] Board the man concerned should be instructed to apply for the pension, and handed a form of application for same.' [79] In January 1917 the Treasury advised that every soldier with mental illness would be entitled to a war pension of thirty shillings per week. If he were 'hospitalised' the man's pension would be distributed so that the relevant state would receive one pound for his keep, while ten shillings would be available either to the soldier's dependants or kept for him until he was discharged from the institution. The states had indicated that they would carry the cost of anything over the one pound per week Commonwealth allowance.[80]

Although there was concern that only genuine cases should receive a pension there was not the same Dickensian approach often remarked upon in the British experience.[81] Private C of the 4th Battalion had been discharged from the AIF on 30 October 1917 and his incapacity (from an unspecified mental illness) was assessed at 50 per cent. Some months later, in March 1918, he was admitted to Callan Park in Sydney where the Master in Lunacy appropriated his pension. Consequently his wife was left almost destitute. A request was made that he be 'taken on the strength of No.13 AAH (Broughton Hall) from the date of his admission to Callan Park so that his costs were covered by the army, and his wife could draw on his pension entitlement. Consequently while he was at Callan Park his incapacity was upgraded to 100 per cent incapacity for the period he was in hospital.'[82]

The reference to a pension (in whatever form) in the medical, military and political literature of the time and indeed through to the thirties, testified to its importance in Australian society and, of course, to the individual concerned. By the twenties the word 'Repat' (a catch-all for both the Repatriation Department, its hospitals and bureaucracy) had entered the nation's folk lexicon. Some saw pensions as a way to successful rehabilitation through offering hope. An influential British psychiatrist believed that 'no patient should be discharged from the Army till cured. It is cruel to send these men back to civilian life unless they have a good post, or a small pension.'[83] Others, however, saw in pensions a reward for as yet unmasked malingerers and that, even in bone fide cases, such monetary compensation would provide a disincentive to self-help. But there was no doubting the longer term effects of war. This was recognised by 1922 in the terms 'exacerbations of a severe type' or 'aggravation' in compensation terminology. 'Just as the concept of "entitlement" dominated early phases of eligibility for pensions and medical treatment, aggravation was instrumental in the evolution of repatriation practice during the 1920s.'[84] More will be said about monetary compensation in the next chapter.

New Directions

While it is not true, at least in the immediate aftermath of the war, that the mental health problems of ex-servicemen were 'swept under the carpet', the future looked bleak in the face of tentative steps to address some of the issues which shell shock indirectly had exposed. Despite a 'general shift in attitude and approach, there was no new consensus among psychiatrists and physicians concerning the phenomenon of shell-shock.'[85] In the early twenties there was certainly sympathy and goodwill, not to mention the significant political clout of veterans' lobby groups, to push for asylum reform and a fair deal for the mentally afflicted 'digger'. But time, increasing political conservatism, and a worsening economic climate would conspire against the shell-shocked and neurotic detritus of the war.

The first significant postwar medical assembly in Australia was the Australasian Medical Congress held in Brisbane in 1920. Traditionally all of the specialist groups reported on their own meetings under its aegis. That year the neurology section adopted several important resolutions that collectively began to place psychology on a more professional footing while also recognising its contribution to medicine. Key recommendations included that 'the universities be asked to provide instruction in psychology for medical students'; and that 'research should be instituted into the aetiology and treatment of the psycho-neuroses and allied mental conditions'. A further recommendation was that in each of 'the capital cities special hospitals should be established for the treatment in the early stages (without certification) of psycho-neurotic and border-line mental conditions.'[86] In writing his medical history of the war, Butler concluded that the wartime experience had led to 'the "humanisation" of the treatment of the insane.'[87] Curiously however, he still believed that 'the study of mentally afflicted soldiers has probably not added to the scientific knowledge of mental disease.' This was despite the fact that he maintained a substantial body of scientific papers on the subject collected after the war to assist him in writing the medical history. Butler's own files include comprehensive medical literature from around the world putting a contrary view.

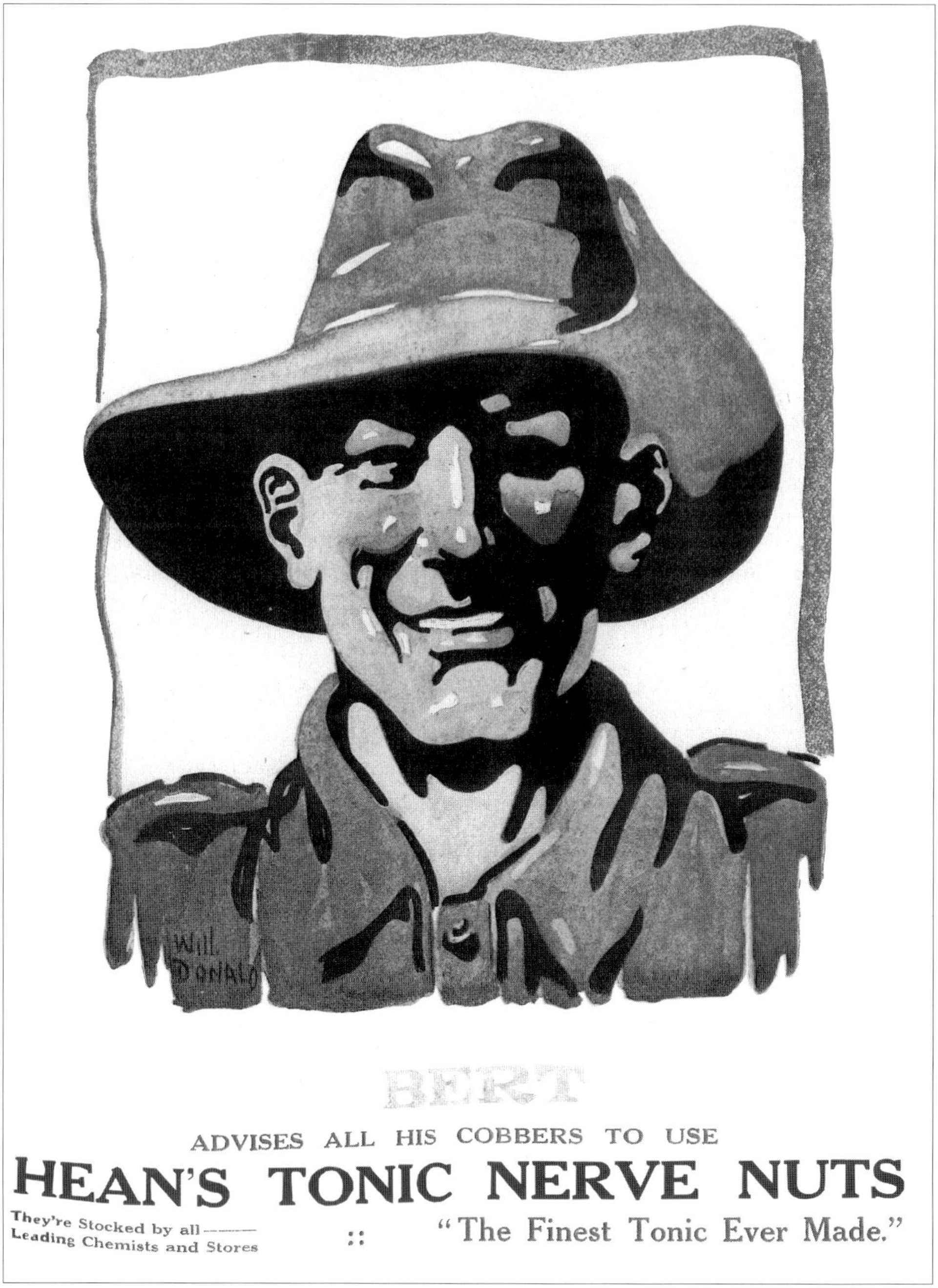
Will Donald
BERT
ADVISES ALL HIS COBBERS TO USE
HEAN'S TONIC NERVE NUTS
They're Stocked by all ——
Leading Chemists and Stores
"The Finest Tonic Ever Made."

While the irony of the product name may have been lost on readers of *Aussie* newspaper, such advertisements for 'cures' were commonplace in the postwar era.
(*Aussie* newspaper)

For Australian psychology the war had actually proved a boon. War neuroses 'stimulated an extensive debate over psychotherapy and its effectiveness.' It seemed that the 'majority of Australian psychiatrists accepted evidence that showed psychotherapy to be effective in the treatment of war neuroses.'[88] Both J. W. Springthorpe and W. Ernest Jones advocated including formal psychology studies in the Australian medical undergraduate curriculum. Shell shock and war neuroses introduced Freudian techniques much faster than would have otherwise occurred, for now doctors 'appropriated and applied—albeit selectively and eclectically—Freudian notions.' This also brought about a shift in treating men with broader mental disorders. 'No longer was it sufficient to look with clinical eyes at men, but psychoanalysis now demanded analytically listening to their language and discourse. The war also produced Australia's first psychoanalysts.'[89] Victoria's Clarence Godfrey, working in No. 5 AGH, was an early proponent of Freudian techniques and he successfully employed hypnosis for the shell-shocked in his care. Some of his colleagues, as we shall see, didn't care for this, preferring either a more disciplined approach or the traditional fare of fresh air and exercise.

Charlatans and others on the periphery or outside orthodox medicine also did well in the immediate postwar years. The popular press of the time was full of pills, tonics and lotions all guaranteed to cure a man of 'nerves'. But some of the pushier quacks resented the short shrift they usually received from officialdom. Since 1909 Mr R. G. Swan (M.P.H.S. Paris) had practised his arts from a Melbourne suburb and his unsmiling face appeared regularly in the pages of newspapers advertising his 'treatment by suggestion'. But in 1918 he felt moved to write a letter to Senator Millen, the Minister for Repatriation. He complained that his approaches to the army had been rebuffed. He was the victim of a conspiracy by the medical profession, a particularly sore point as he was 'the only qualified suggestion specialist in Australia.'[90] The advice to the Minister from his own department was that Swan was not only 'a charlatan of the ordinary type', but he was 'absolutely without standing.'[91] There remains the suspicion, however, that his complaint was not entirely without grounds.

Another important consequence of the war was 'a reorientation of psychiatric theory from a "materialist" basis' which sought to explain abnormal psychological behaviour by positing actual physical changes in the brain or nervous system, towards the recognition that 'neurotic behaviour might be primarily "psychogenic" in nature—resulting from shock, fright or mental conflict rather than physical trauma.'[92] But, from the soldier's point of view, this 'enlightened' progress did not necessarily mean he was relieved of responsibility for his own plight. Analysis had, by definition, at last removed the symptom from the moral area. It could be said that individual neurosis 'was not the result of a conscious decision made by the patient. On the contrary, the neurotic soldier was one who could repudiate neither his desire for survival nor the ideals and moral imperatives that kept him at the front.'[93]

The very public debate about shell shock and the fact that many citizens lived with, or knew of husbands, relatives or friends suffering from war neuroses, did spur a number of developments in postwar Australia. These included improvement in the conditions of treatment which had repercussions in civil practice, and extra-institutional organised endeavours to provide such mental and physical amenities. Unfortunately some of the same lessons had to be relearned after the Second World War, while others such as the stigma of mental disease would return in 1940. Equally significant but more hidden was the war's contribution to the mental suffering and social cost to individuals and their families.

Cured or Cursed?

What did all this mean for those men who were already being treated for neuroses, or for the increasing numbers of ex-servicemen who, as the war receded, began to relive the horrors of war? The official line—that the only people who continued to suffer were those predisposed to mental illness or were neurotically paralysed by pensions—was belied by the observations of many doctors. '...Some of [their ex-soldier patients] had come through unscathed only to break down after demobilisation.'[94] This trend would continue after the war. In the early 1920s an Australian psychologist acknowledged the advances made in the 'psychological knowledge of functional nervous disablement' and the contribution of Sigmund Freud in throwing 'light into some of the most obscure regions of the normal human mind.' He still had to admit, however, that 'the knowledge so far obtained is not as yet widely spread, *nor perhaps, always well understood where it has penetrated* [emphasis added].'[95] If this was the state of the profession, how could the wider society deal with its war-damaged veterans?

It was Dr W. R. Regnell's belief that, without attempting 'any scientific classification of war neuroses, we may divide the cases we are likely to come across into three groups: neurasthenia, hysteria and psychasthenia.'[96] Regnell suggested that most men suffering from hysteria were susceptible to suggestion and made a good recovery. Soldiers labelled 'hysterical' also made up sixty per cent 'of those seen in special neurological hospitals.' But, as we shall see, such optimism was not always vindicated as the war receded in all but the minds of those most affected by it.

Endnotes

1 Butler, *Official History*, vol. III, p. 66.
2 MacPherson et al., *History of the Great War*, vol. II, p. 34.
3 Stone, 'Shellshock and the Psychiatrists', p. 244.
4 Kathleen Jones, *Asylums and After: a Revised History of the Mental Health Services from the Early 18th Century to the Late 1990s*, Athlone, London, 1939.
5 Like every other section of society the civilian health infrastructure had to make sacrifices. Chiefly this took the form of trained personnel joining the services. However many ex-asylum staff also found their way into the military as the latter recognised their particular skills. These staff included officers, nurses and orderlies.
6 Letter to Headquarters 2nd Military District (New South Wales) from the medical officer at No. 3 AAH (Broughton Hall) 11 December 1915 concerning orderlies. File: 14/8979. Broughton Hall Correspondence. State Records of New South Wales.
7 Leese, 'Why are they not cured?', p. 209.
8 Thomson, 'Status, Manpower and Mental Fitness', p.154.
9 Butler, *Official History*, vol. III, pages 882 and 939.
10 M. J. Lewis, *Managing Madness: psychiatry and society in Australia 1788–1980*, AGPS Press, Canberra, 1988, p. 36.
11 Butler, *Official History*, vol. II, p. 74.
12 Susan Fennell, 'Psychiatry in New Zealand 1912–1948' in B. Brookes and J. Thomson (eds.), *Unfortunate Folk: Essays on Mental Health Trends in New Zealand 1863–1992*, University of Otago, 2001, p. 145.
13 Damousi, *Freud*, p. 49.
14 Bogacz, 'War Neurosis and Cultural Change in England 1914–1922', p. 31.
15 Ibid., p. 29.
16 Downey, 'The Management and Treatment of Early Insanity', p. 719.
17 Letter from the Secretary of the Defence Department to the Secretary of the Repatriation Department, 15 October 1917. AWM 253 AIF 498/1/693.
18 Mental Hospitals—AAMC Conference, Director General of Medical Services. Minutes of DGMS Conference 17 June 1918. AWM 25 /399/18/213.
19 A 2487/1/1921/9338. Newspaper Clippings, National Archives Australia (Canberra).
20 The New Zealand experience in this regard was not dissimilar. Patriotic associations there 'pressured officials into distorting the legal committal process to mental hospitals, established novel types of institutions for soldiers, and experimented with new and less stigmatising psychiatric labels.' John Weaver and David Wright, 'Shell Shock and the Politics of Asylum Committal in New Zealand, 1916–1922', *Heath and History*, vol. 7, no.1, 2005, p.19.
21 Letter from the Inspector General of the Insane, Victoria, to the Minister for Defence, 30 November 1917. AAMC Units in Australia—Special Hospitals Mental, Mont Park Victoria, AWM 32 [63].
22 Letter from the Secretary of the Defence Department to the Secretary of the Repatriation Department, 15 October 1917. AWM 253 AIF 498/1/693.
23 AAMC Units in Australia, Special Hospitals, Mental—General File, AWM 32 [61].
24 Ibid.
25 W. Ernest Jones (Victorian Inspector General of the Insane) report, Mont Park, Heidelberg, Victoria, August 1917. Mental Hospitals, AWM 25 /399/18/213.
26 No.13 AAH, Mental Hospitals. AWM 25 /399/18/213.
27 Stephen Garton, *Medicine and Madness: A Social History of Insanity in New South Wales 1880-1940*, University of New South Wales Press, Sydney, 1988, pp.153–4.
28 In this it reflected general military practice whereby in general hospitals officers were usually segregated from other ranks.

29 For example Clarence Godfrey, a leading advocate of hypnosis, could still write in 1918 that many soldiers in his care 'had a definite neurotic history.' 'Some Cases of Stammering from War Shock treated by Psychotherapy', *MJA*, 28 September 1918, p. 262.
30 Regnell, 'The Psychoneuroses of War', p. 457.
31 Leese, 'Why are they not cured?', pp. 217–18.
32 Shepherd, *A War of Nerves*, p. 50. Myers left the front in November 1917, 'frustrated and exhausted by day-to-day struggles with prejudice and ignorance...' W. Holden, *Shell Shock*, Channel 4 Books, London, 1998, p. 46.
33 Showalter, *The Female Malady*, p. 176.
34 E. D. Adrian and L. R. Yealland, 'Treatment of Some Common War Neuroses', *Lancet*, 9 June 1917, p. 870.
35 Showalter, *The Female Malady*, p. 177.
36 Adrian and Yealland, 'Treatment of Some Common War Neuroses', p. 869.
37 P. Dane, 'Traumatic Psychoneurosis', *MJA*, 25 February 1950, p. 267.
38 Adrian and Yealland, 'Treatment of Some Common War Neuroses', p. 868.
39 Leed, *No Man's Land*, p. 171.
40 Garton, *Medicine and Madness*, p. 157.
41 Stone, 'Shellshock and the Psychiatrists', p. 255.
42 Oppenheim, *Shattered Nerves*, p. 309.
43 Regnell, 'The Psychoneuroses of War', p. 458.
44 Merskey, 'Shell-Shock', p. 247.
45 Garton, *Medicine and Madness*, p. 160.
46 Merskey, 'Shell-Shock', p. 245.
47 Springthorpe, 'War Neuroses and Civil Practice', p. 280
48 Damousi, *Freud in the Antipodes*, p. 51.
49 Ibid., pages 50 and 51.
50 Paul Dane, 'The Psycho-Neuroses of Soldiers and their Treatment' in *MJA*, 25 April 1925, p. 429.
51 MacPherson, et al., *History of the Great War*, vol. II, p. 65.
52 Stone, 'Shellshock and the Psychiatrists', p. 247.
53 *Report of the Shell Shock Commission*, HMSO, London, 1922, p. 144.
54 Bogacz, 'War Neurosis and Cultural Change in England 1914–1922', p. 48.
55 Leese, 'Why are they not cured?', p. 143.
56 Peter Barham, *Forgotten Lunatics of the Great War*, Yale Press, London, 2004, p. 233.
57 Jones, 'Case of Shell Shock', p. 203.
58 Feudtner, 'Minds the Dead Have Ravished', p. 389.
59 Leed, *No Man's Land*, p. 170.
60 Butler, for example, in a reference to homosexuality in Magnus Hirshfield's *Sexual History of the War*, called it 'an unpleasant book.' Butler, *Official History*, vol. III, p. 137.
61 Lewis, *Managing Madness*, p. 39.
62 Letter from the Secretary of the Defence Department to the Secretary of the Repatriation Department, 15 October 1917. AWM 253 AIF 498/1/693.
63 Lewis, *Managing Madness*, p. 39.
64 Memorandum from Secretary of the Defence Department to the Secretary of the Repatriation Department, 29 October 1917. 'Mental Hospitals'. AWM 25 /399/18/213.
65 Mental Hospitals—AAMC Conference, Director General of Medical Services. Minutes of DGMS Conference 17 June 1918. AWM 25 /399/18/213.
66 Letter, 15 September 1920. A2489.20/1447. NAA (Canberra).
67 Report on Observations of Invalid Boards by Colonel Sir Harry Maudsley, September 1918, p. 8. AWM 27 376/24.
68 File: 14/8963. State Records of New South Wales.
69 *MJA*, 3 May 1919, p. 367.
70 File: 14/8956. State Records of New South Wales.

71 No.16 AGH, Macleod, Victoria, Report 30 June 1918. AWM 3 DRL 32/20.
72 Despite the lessons learned from 1915 to 1918, the predisposition theory would regain centre place in the repatriation bureaucracy of the Second World War.
73 Eder, *War Shock*, p. 144.
74 Raftery, *Marks of War*, p. 21.
75 Major S.V. Sewel, 'Mental Hospitals—AAMC Conference, Director General of Medical Services'. Minutes of DGMS Conference, 17 June 1918. AWM 25 /399/18/213.
76 Report: 'The Treatment of "Neurasthenia" in Soldiers', *MJA*, 7 December 1918, p. 481.
77 MacPherson et al., *History of the Great War*, vol. II, p. 35.
78 Raftery, *Marks of War*, p. 17.
79 Broughton Hall Correspondence, Letter of February 1916, File: 14/8979. State Records of New South Wales.
80 Treasury advice to the Prime Minister's office, 24 January 1917. AIF 498/1/693. AWM.
81 For Australian concerns see Tyquin, *Gallipoli: the Medical War* and for the situation in Britain see Barham's *Forgotten Lunatics of the Great War*.
82 File: 14/8959. State Records of New South Wales.
83 Eder, *War Shock*, p. 143.
84 Clem Lloyd and J. Rees, *The Last Shilling: A History of Repatriation in Australia*, Melbourne University Press, 1994, p. 228.
85 Deane, *Shook Over Hell*, p. 33.
86 *MJA*, 18 September 1920, p. 303.
87 Butler, *Official History*, vol. III., p. 835.
88 Garton, *Medicine and Madness*, p. 82.
89 Damousi, *Freud in the Antipodes*, p. 33.
90 Letter, 30 December 1918. A.2489.20/1447 NAA (Canberra).
91 Memorandum, 4 January1919. A.2489.20/1447 NAA (Canberra).
92 Deane, *Shook Over Hell*, p. 33.
93 Leed, *No Man's Land*, p. 176.
94 Shepherd, *A War of Nerves*, p. 152.
95 Lowson, 'Some Points in the Psychology of Nervous Breakdown', p. 113.
96 Regnell, 'The Psychoneuroses of War', p. 455.

Chapter Seven
Civilian Life: a Cold, Disappointing Thing?

It must have been disappointing for some neurotic soldiers to find the task of fitting back into civilian life was far more challenging than they had expected. No doubt some found it too hard and joined society's detritus in the street gutters or the haunts of the 'metho' drinkers. Some of the public too found it hard to associate soldiers' experiences in the war with their eccentric or even anti-social behaviour. It would have unnerved the nation to come face-to-face with the unexpected prevalence of shell-shocked men in its midst—surely a threat to public health? For those families caught in the middle it could be a sad time as they struggled with pensions legislation and the erring ways of loved ones, while the state thrashed out financial arrangements and the Repatriation Commission increasingly took on the role of custodian of the nation's military mad.

Governments have argued that a certain proportion of the psychological fall-out of the war would have occurred anyway. As the *British Official History* made clear, most of these men could not, in any case, have made a successful adaptation to the conditions of postwar life, and there can be little doubt that, in its view, even had there been no war, these men would sooner or later, and from one cause or another, have been likely to break down under the stress of everyday life.[1] 'Those left, all this suggests, were not "war neurotics", just neurotics and mental weaklings...Increasingly a moralistic, judgmental tone emerged.'[2] This was pretty much the tone adopted by Butler in his *Official History*. His attitude may have been fashioned partly by his direct experience of the large numbers of mentally unfit who had managed to enlist or who were later prevented from joining the army. However both these 'official' historians subtly distanced their respective nations from any recognition of the realities of neuroses in war by suggesting that many of the men were, to all intents and purposes, mad anyway. So for much of the early postwar period it fell to ex-soldiers' associations to fight a rearguard action against the perception that their colleagues deserved nothing of the adulation accorded to the majority of AIF members by a grateful nation.

As discussed previously, there were a number of differences between Australia and Britain in the treatment of, and approach to, shell shock. Looking at the management of neurotic soldiers after the war, a key distinction lies in the fact that British veterans' movements 'played no significant part in interwar political life.'[3] In addition, while both governments shared a concern over the legitimacy of some pensions on the grounds of mental illness from war service, the Australian approach was generally more sympathetic in the day-to-day administration of the shell-shocked. Nor was there in Australia the legacy of pauper asylums still found in the United Kingdom and, unlike the English experience, there was real development in the civil asylum system. This continued until the end of the decade when the Great Depression would push more ex-servicemen 'over the edge' and financial constraints would see a number of civilian asylums squeezed for finances. Australia too was still largely an agrarian-based economy and had not the same sophisticated network of worker's compensation and insurance, with its concomitant clinical baggage, as was the case in the United Kingdom, Germany and the United States. However, despite the progress of psychology in society generally, the place of hysteria and hereditary predisposition still lingered in postwar Australia, especially in the medical profession.

In spite of better mental health care and the growing time-span since the war, the problems of the neurotic soldier did not go away. Alistair Thompson, in his interviews with Australian survivors of that war noted with surprise that there 'was a staggering incidence of mental disorder among returned diggers.' All his interviewees had vivid stories about soldier friends 'who went crazy, became derelict drunks or killed themselves.'[4] Families were affected, if not fractured, and although society was keen to move on, at this time it still felt a sense of obligation to these men, an attitude that would dissipate through the twenties. With increasing frequency, newspapers reported neurotic ex-servicemen running amok and committing crimes. By the mid-1920s there was a curious vacillation of public opinion in Australia when it came to ex-servicemen with war neuroses. Of Britain it has been said that there was a striking contrast between 'prevailing military and medical attitudes' to shell shock and those held by 'the parliament, the newspapers and the public at large.'[5] This pattern was largely mirrored in Australia. For the public, at least in the short term, the mood was best expressed by a newspaper editorial typical of the time:

> ...there are these youths who left homes of peace and comfort for the hardships of war and all its attendant horrors, and the stress on brain and mind have been enormous. For many of them life will never be the same again...many who have returned have found that, after the first enthusiastic welcome home, life could be a cold, disappointing thing.[6]

There was also the total inability of the nation's citizens to understand or relate to the worst experiences suffered by those of its soldiers who had been at the front. This is probably true of all wars, but the insulation imposed by distance played a bigger role for Australia. If a sullen soldiery perplexed the denizens of London, a few kilometres from the Western Front, Australians had even less chance of comprehending their shattered menfolk. After all, the public was 'weary of war, recoiling from its horror, and sickened by the number of its victims, tried to forget those tragic years as quickly as possible.' Bill Gammage, in his appositely titled *The Broken Years*, makes the point that civilians 'were unable or unwilling to comprehend either the magnitude of the soldier's ordeal, or the force of the memories, good and bad, which separated returned men from others. They wanted a return to normalcy, and they expected returned men to show a similar desire.'[7] As we have seen this was probably a tall order.

It was this unrealistic expectation that proved to be the main cause of the progressive loss of public sympathy for the military's mad. This impatience with war neurotics would carry over into the public commemoration of that war which, after the thirties, was being cemented into the social fabric of Australia.[8] The other challenge was that no-one really knew how long the effects of shell shock would last, nor what the costs to the community would be. Psychologists such as Elton Mayo, who lectured in philosophy at the University of Queensland during the war, believed firmly that shell shock remained long after the event. This had been the source of many disputes, and Freud himself believed that war neurosis would end with the Armistice. 'But one of the cruel lessons of the war was the fact that shell shock did endure.'[9]

Despite the still fresh horrors of war, even some doctors were sceptical. Public compassion had its limits and could not be sustained through to the 1930s with the same vigour it had shown in the early twenties. The medical officer who accompanied the last contingent of seventy psychiatric patients from Europe, Captain Oliver Latham, admitted that he had had a good opportunity to examine them on board ship during the long, tedious voyage home. He noted that many of 'the true psychoses were of such a nature and occurred in physical types that suggested these people were *doomed* to *insanity* no matter what life they had taken up.' He went on to list the Elysian picture army life meant—free food, shelter etc. He then came out with this extraordinary (to our eyes) pronouncement:

> You will see on the part of the Private and in some respects in the Officer section a freedom from financial and unhappy family cares of the most remarkable order—why, many a potential psychotic was kept free from mental ill-health for quite a

time, to *fail* [emphasis added] when conditions became too strenuous or *when he came back full grown to full responsible manhood* and having to face the world against all comers.[10]

Pensions

While it had sent troops to the second Anglo-Boer War at the turn of the century, Australia had no system of military pensioning before World War I. Subsequently the Commonwealth Government passed the *War Pensions Act* on 21 December 1914, four years before the British Government established its Ministry of Pensions. A raft of further legislation in the early twenties followed. In Australia the Act established a framework within which all soldiers, including those with war-related injuries, physical or mental, could seek support if they were unemployable or too ill. Nurses and other female service personnel, however, had a much harder struggle to make a case for their claims.[11] Under the Australian system the attribution of any damage to military service was classified either as 'due to war service' or 'due to war service and aggravation'. As such it was quite distinct from the system in other countries after the war. The nation's commitment to pension and treatment regimes (with the possible exception of the US) 'exceeded, in proportion both to troops engaged and to population, those of any other nation.'[12]

The Act was administered first by the Defence Department and later by the newly formed Repatriation Department. Much of the postwar military and medical machinery went into overseeing the burgeoning claims made on the pensions system, which was quite elaborate, with a carefully calibrated system of compensation for missing body parts, blindness, deafness and other disabilities. In Britain shell shock 'was second only to wounds in the pensions awards list for the First World War.'[13] By comparison, in Australia in 1924 there were 72,760 persons registered as war pensioners of whom four per cent were 'mental cases'. By 1939 the total figure had risen to 77,151, and of this, larger figure, five per cent were classified as having psychological problems.[14]

Military authorities in Australia had about eight weeks' warning by cable of the number of psychiatric patients returning home from abroad. Lists were classified by state and once ships reached the first port of call (Fremantle in Western Australia) detailed information was relayed regarding the nature of the casualties and the identity of the patients. After disembarking from their special transports or troop-ships, soldiers diagnosed with psychological problems went before a medical board which determined whether they would be returned to duty, referred for specialist treatment or discharged unfit. Soldiers were then advised to go before the Pensions Department in their own state to see if they were eligible for a pension.

However this 'system' evolved slowly in an ad hoc fashion with variations in procedures between the states. From 1914 to 1917 each state was still largely a 'law unto itself" and a very wide discrepancy in practice grew up, 'especially as to whether these cases should be treated under military control or discharged early to civilian treatment.' At first they were taken into general hospitals without any actual discrimination. In New South Wales and Victoria, mainly on the initiative of the state Mental Departments, an attempt was made to segregate them under specialist treatment. But 'speaking generally there is no evidence that the Defence Department seriously grappled with the problem until 1918, when big reforms were initiated in every branch of finalising treatment.'[15]

Until the Armistice in 1918 the various states cared for all those ex-servicemen not in military hospitals. 'Those who had not been cured within 12 months were sent back to their respective state lunacy departments. At this time all mentally disturbed citizens were subject to state statutes that determined how they were treated and housed.'[16] The Director General of Medical Services in Australia, Major-General Richard Fetherston, recommended that those certified insane, after discharge from the AIF, be handed over to the various state Lunacy Departments, the cost of their maintenance to be a charge against the soldier's pension. This same arrangement was hugely unpopular in Britain and caused anxiety for not a few families in Australia.

A worried mother wrote to the Minister for Repatriation in Melbourne: 'I am sorry to have to inform you that Jack is in Callan Park Asylum, [war] wounds and drink being the cause. I was told when visiting at the mental hospital by the doctor and attendants and Jack himself that returned soldiers have special food provided by the Red Cross...Now this being so, how is it that the Master in Lunacy proposed to claim his pension for his keep?' She understood that patients' pensions, as in the case of her son, were exempt from payment to institutions.[17] She subsequently received a telegram from the Minister stating that this was not the case. However, in her second letter she noted that 'a number of soldier patients who had no relatives needed visitors as well as some reassurance that they were not to lose their pensions.'[18] This letter, addressed directly to the Minister, is not untypical of the time and indicates either the writer's frustration with the bureaucracy or a misunderstanding of how the legislation was supposed to work.

There evolved then clear policy guidelines for all treating military hospitals with respect to eligibility for pensions. At Broughton Hall, for instance, patients presented with acute or chronic psychiatric symptoms. Those with the latter were simply discharged and pensioned from the army to be eventually 'picked up' by the state systems. If it were proven that their problems were not the result of military service, these men were advised to enter an asylum (and the majority of admissions were voluntary), thereby releasing the Commonwealth from the financial burden of paying for their hospital accommodation. In the event that a soldier's condition was clearly the result of, or aggravated by, his war service, then he remained at Broughton Hall (whose treatment regime included suggestion, persuasion and the 'free association' methods then in vogue) until he recovered, or if this did not occur, indefinitely, with a view to avoiding certification under the state lunacy laws. Military doctors were aware that if a patient left the army and was pensioned, even though he required ongoing treatment, he could not be retained under army regulations, 'however acute the mental symptoms might be'. In this case neurotic soldiers would leave Broughton Hall and many not submit to treatment, although (if their condition did not improve or they had not suicided) there was a strong possibility that they would eventually gravitate to civilian asylums.

According to its superintendent, the main objective in pensioning soldiers off 'appears to be the reduction in the expense by the difference between the amount of pension and pay.' He saw an advantage in being able to prevent returned soldiers, whose illness was a direct result of active service, from being certified and sent to a mental hospital as an ordinary insane patient—enough in his opinion 'to justify the expense.' It was therefore necessary that the patient should remain a member of the AIF so that 'the treating doctors maintained their authority as his military superior' with the aim of curing him before letting him fend for himself.[19] It was an unashamedly paternalistic approach and illustrated the importance of power in doctor-patient relationships which, especially in the mental health sphere, has been commented upon in much of the literature on shell shock.

In 1916 the responsibility for determining pensions had been handed to military medical officers, and 'boards' of two such officers were set up around the country. While the Commonwealth Treasury administered all war pensions until 1920, mental patients continued to be dealt with by the various states. But the irascible John Springthorpe was furious at the reception some patients received. He knew that some 'were treated as malingerers and discharged without army pensions to come up for reconsideration and necessary treatment after many months of dissatisfaction.' This left a number to fend for themselves, trying to fit into 'environments for which they were unfitted, largely without any guiding and suitable line of treatment.' Acknowledging the part of pensions in postwar society, he contended that many ex-servicemen were still 'in an unsatisfactory condition, partly perhaps because their future remains unsettled, but more from want of recognition of their psychology and continued neglect of its requirements.'[20] While the Australian war pension system did not automatically grant all returned soldiers a pension, it is not true to say, as some have done, that 'if a returned digger had some chance of receiving a pension and medical treatment for a war wound, he had almost no chance of getting any official support for psychological damage.'[21]

However suspicion of malingering and 'not playing the game' lingered in official circles. Even in his official history Butler could not avoid espousing his prejudices. He followed convention by linking moral and mental disorders and went on to say that in pension claimants '*entitlement* and *treatment* are so inextricably inter-related as to make them in effect, a single medical issue and, only too often, a "vicious circle."' Butler conjoined the two conditions by referring to 'burnt out' or 'war-worn' soldiers, whom he believed were a legitimate group. But here his sympathy stopped, as he believed that for the mentally ill soldier 'the mind must heal itself and a man must heal his own mind.'[22] The reasons are not hard to find. 'War was the supreme test of manliness, and those who were the victims of shell shock had failed this test. But, in as much as the manly ideal reflected the norms established society had set for itself, the shell-shocked soldier bore not only the burden of his sickness; he had also left the confines of normal society and taken on the image common to outsiders.'[23] This seems to fit with Charles Bean's own perception of war as the ultimate forge of nations. Secondly, his vision for the country was gathering momentum and it was supported at all levels of Australian society from the ex-commanders now in positions of power in the parliaments, industry, agriculture and the judiciary, to the ex-diggers, now formalising their own memories of the war and seeing themselves, not always with justification, in the role of warrior heroes. As the war receded, however, Australian society took on a more disapproving attitude to its 'mad' veterans.

Government Financial Arrangements

In September 1917 the Federal Parliament passed the *Australian Soldiers' Repatriation Act* which came into law on 8 April 1918. In 1920, under pressure from ex-service associations, this was amended by another act and a Commonwealth Minister for Repatriation (Sir Neville Howse VC, former head of the AAMC) was appointed.[24] But the sovereign rights of the states bedevilled the system. Responsibility for treating soldiers with mental illness remained with the Defence Department until 1921, the Repatriation Department only taking over once soldiers were discharged from the military hospitals, although that department did help fund such hospitals. The early history of the Repatriation Commission and the Department was embroiled in claims that it was either biased or not doing enough for returned soldiers. This led to a Royal Commission (consisting, significantly, of five doctors) into its activities in 1924, with a brief to investigate how war service disabilities (including psychological problems) were assessed. A major problem was the lack of detailed medical records, the destruction of which was referred to previously. The system was revisited in 1929 with the formation of appeals assessment tribunals. In their first year of operation they dealt with 2,915 appeals (of which 1,382 were rejected).[25]

As in peace, there was little sacred in war, and the issue of unbalanced returned servicemen became a political football for the next two decades, feeding off the real or imagined concerns of soldiers' relatives and friends and political opportunists. In November 1917 Sir John Forrest (Leader of the Federal Opposition) telegrammed the Minister for Defence, Senator George Pearce (also from Western Australia). Forrest informed him that he had 'passed legislation arranging for treatment of mentally deranged soldiers without certification.' The Prime Minister had already been told in May that the small number of returned mental casualties from that state did not 'warrant establishment [of] separate institutions.' The telegram stated that four mentally deranged soldiers were receiving treatment at Claremont Lunatic Asylum near Perth. Their relatives, official lunacy visitors, and other returned soldiers were protesting against this decision. Consequently the State Labor (opposition) Party was 'using it as a cry against the National Party in the Subiaco [a Perth suburb] by-election, and will use it in the conscription campaign.'[26]

All state authorities did their best to cooperate with the Commonwealth Government in providing accommodation and special care, but the relationship was prone to constant public criticism. The challenge of representing the neurotic soldier was taken up largely by ex-service organisations. However, perhaps driven by misguided enthusiasm, other agencies such as *Smith's Weekly*, a Sydney-based threepenny populist newspaper, continued to champion the cause throughout the 1920s and 1930s, especially in its 'Sailors' and Soldiers' Parliament' column, irrespective of the merits of individual cases.[27] But it was not always wrong. For example in 1926 'it was able to point out that 8,000 Diggers were dying each year at an average age of forty-five' some from mental illness.[28] There was never any love lost between this newspaper and the Repatriation Commission which the newspaper dubbed in 1921 the 'Cyanide Gang.'[29]

Returned Sailors and Soldiers' Imperial League of Australia

(NEW SOUTH WALES BRANCH)

Hospital Entertainment & Welfare Committee

LONE MENTAL DIGGERS' FUND.

H. P. ASHBURNER, CHAIRMAN.
W. E. DOMAN, HON. SEC.
W. W. MILES, HON. TREAS.
S. MURRAY, HON. PUBLICITY OFFICER.

Anzac Memorial,
Hyde Park, Sydney.
1st August, 1936.

Dear Sir or Madam:

The Great War of 1914-1918 has been responsible for no more tragic result than the breaking down of the mental resistance of so many ex-servicemen. Many hundreds of them are domiciled in the various mental homes and asylums in New South Wales, and their plight is causing grave concern to the State Branch of the R.S.S.I.L.A., which has approved of the care of such cases being undertaken by the Hospital Entertainment and Welfare Committee.

The majority of the hospital patients with physical disabilities, even those who are permanently or semi-permanently inmates of the Repatriation and Red Cross Hospitals are in receipt of military pension or sustenance, and of a measure of comfort to off-set, in some small degree, the terrific price they are paying for service in their country's need. But the Mental Case — What of him?

Do you realise that, in Callan Park Mental Asylum alone, there are over 200 ex-servicemen, the great majority of them without Military pension because war causage has not yet been proven.

They are in urgent need of such small comforts as cigarettes, tobacco, etc., and this Committee is resolved that they shall not so want.

FUNDS, HOWEVER, ARE URGENTLY NEEDED!

To provide 1oz. tobacco with cigarette papers, or an equivalent issue of cigarettes to each pensionless patient in Callan Park alone will cost approximately £10 each week. Add to this the needs of the other nine Mental Institutions in N.S.W., and some idea will be obtained of the magnitude of the undertaking.

Here are the views of some of the "Men who know":—

L. A. Robb Esq., C.M.G., State President of the R.S.S.I.L.A., says:

"The case of the Mental ex-servicemen is indeed a tragic one. I know of no more pressing need than the provision of smokes for these terribly afflicted comrades of ours . . . . Good luck to the Hospital Entertainment and Welfare Committee, and may God speed their efforts on behalf of these unfortunate ex-servicemen."

Capt. G. D. Mitchell, M.C., D.C.M., Author of the powerful articles on war-time and post-war subjects appearing in "Reveille":

"I was invited to Callan Park to see for myself. I went . . . . I saw . . . . and was shaken to the very depths of my being! My one ambition now is to assist in bringing some little sunshine to these ex-servicemen, and I am happy to take my place on the Committee that I might add my weight to the work in hand . . . ."

Capt. C. T. Agassiz ("Aggy")—The popular Hospital Cheerio Man of 2UE:

"Whilst I visit thousands of patients in the various Hospitals every year, I come across many lonely ex-servicemen who, through sickness, pain, worry and anxiety, are absolutely in the 'Depths of Misery'. In most cases, a few comforts in the shape of sweets, fruit and tobacco have greatly assisted in bucking them up. A cheery word and a handshake never fail to bring them to the realisation that someone cares for the 'digger who did his bit'.

"No visit to any institution has ever touched me so much as that to *Callan Park Mental Asylum*. There are housed in various Mental Asylums hundreds of men who were good soldiers—men who went through all that you and I did, and because their faculties could not stand the strain, they are cast aside to spend their declining years as virtual prisoners.

"We must never let it be said that these lonely diggers are allowed to languish without the little comforts which so assist, at least, to recompense them for an existence which is comparable with prison life—without the armed warder.

"Funds are necessary, promptness is advisable, and no man stands straighter than when he stoops to help a friend."

YOUR GENEROUS SUPPORT IS SOLICITED!

All donations will be acknowledged through the "Daily Telegraph" and in "Reveille," the official organ of the R.S.S.I.L.A.

Kindly make your remittances to—

W. W. MILES, Hon. Treas.,
Anzac Memorial, Hyde Park,
Sydney.

With thanks for your anticipated co-operation,

Yours faithfully,
W. E. DOMAN,
Hon. Secretary.

ADDRESS ALL CORRESPONDENCE TO
BOX 37 P.O., GEORGE STREET NORTH,
SYDNEY

Pleas such as these from lobby groups who felt a special responsibility for the war neurotics became commonplace through the 1930s. (National Archives of Australia. SP 459/1, 471/1/299)

Interestingly, the other popular soldiers' magazine, *Aussie* (begun in France in 1918 and which continued until 1932) provided more humour and sentimentality and published some telling amateur poetry that was rather more revealing than Bean would ever accept for his material. But it never took on the adversarial role that *Smith's Weekly* obviously savoured. Another paper *The Australian Worker* also had the government in its sights and, by 1917, was railing against the 'maudlin patriotism' of politicians and the mainstream press while they ignored the plight of returning soldiers.

Relations between federal and state agencies continued to be criticised by the ex-service lobby. It believed, often without solid grounds, that only the Commonwealth could deliver the best treatment to the war neurotic. At one large meeting of the Returned Sailors' and Soldiers' League there was strong 'condemnation of the present method of treatment of returned soldier mental cases.' In fact the gathering was 'unanimous that the care of mental cases was the duty of the Commonwealth and not of the State.' As one member of the executive put it, 'of all the men who were suffering from the effects of the war, no-one needed more careful consideration and attention than the mentally afflicted. Effective segregation was also a necessity.' He believed that this system of segregation would lead to the ultimately successful restoration of the individual to society.[30] Richard Fetherston (now out of uniform and practising once more as a civilian doctor) said that it was imperative that the war cases not be passed into civilian hospitals. 'These patients must be cared for as though they were still soldiers.'

Various financial arrangements were put in place during the war and this example from Victoria is not untypical. Early in 1918 the state's Inspector General of the Insane informed the Medical Superintendent at Royal Park that he had arranged with the Repatriation Board that it 'pay at the rate of 30/- per week for the maintenance of each patient under care from the date of his discharge from the Military Forces until his discharge' from Mont Park. If, subsequently, any ex-soldier was 'committed under the Lunacy Act to the Hospital for the Insane, the Master will collect the amount due', but the Defence Department would collect it while the patient was cared for under the *Mental Treatment Act*.[31] In other words the Defence Department was liable for payments to the asylum up to the date of the soldier's discharge from the AIF. Reference has already been made to the separate 'deals' between the Commonwealth and the states for the accommodation and treatment of soldiers and to arrange payment for these resources.

In another example, at Stromness in Western Australia, the Repatriation Commission had concluded an agreement with that state's government to pay

£150 per annum for the services of its Inspector General of the Insane, in addition to paying for asylum employees, maintenance, and for the patients there.[32] Even during the war there were very few exclusively military asylums, and even these often also catered for tuberculous and other patients who needed to be segregated on medical grounds. These institutions were: No. 16 AGH (Mont Park) in Heidelberg, Victoria; No. 13 AAH (Broughton Hall); No. 28 AAH in Leichhardt, New South Wales; and No. 24 AAH, Cottesloe, in Western Australia. Soldiers from Queensland were sent to Goodna or later, to Toowoomba, while those from Tasmania were sent to New Norfolk.

In 1943 Butler listed the courses of treatment by the Repatriation Commission for both its in-patients and out-patients. Patient types were listed as: 'War Neurosis, including Epileptics, Neurasthenics, Shell Shocks, Alcoholics and Inebriates.'[33] It is also interesting to note that even he was still using the phrase 'shell shock'. According to his figures, the number of patients suffering war neuroses in 1922 had totalled 1,885, a figure that climbed slowly until 1927 when 1,926 soldiers were receiving treatment. By 1936 the number had climbed further to 3,819 and by 1939 it had reached 4,891—and these were only the 'reported' cases known to the authorities. The incidence of mental illness among the ex-service population now provoked the same polarity that shell shock had during the war. There were those who saw neuroses as a legitimate medical condition and those who could discern the sinister shadow of malingering in every mental case.

In January 1927 Sir Philip Gibbs, a former wartime journalist, wrote an open letter to the British *Overseas* magazine titled: 'Wounded Souls—A Plea for Nerve-Strained Victims of the War.' In the margin of a copy of this article Butler scribbled 'appalling muck'.[34] Dr E. L. Forward, the chief medical inspector of the British Ministry of Pensions, rebutted in detail much of Gibbs's argument. Both Butler and Forward seem to have missed the point, for although the language was melodramatic, part of Gibbs's article was prescient as far as some of these afflicted men were concerned. He referred to 'thousands of British homes [in which] there have been these tragedies, pitiable beyond all words, because they have been suffered in loneliness, in the agony of long-waking nights, with secret fears hidden even from wives and mothers who knew these men when they were gay lads, before the War.'[35] Despite the pleading there was truth in the prose. There is no doubt that the lives of some who survived the war would be shattered forever, a prediction shared by others. The Australian *Repatriation* magazine published an article by an American officer titled 'Invisible Wounds'. Referring to the American public, he said that the shell-shocked 'must not be passed by because their sacrifices are not obvious, they must be given full opportunity to regain their positions in life.'[36] Despite claims to the contrary, there was, in the immediate postwar years, a very real and genuine effort on the part of both the army and the government to do its best by these men in Australia.

Saints to Sinners

The first indication that not all was well with some returned soldiers was seen in the home. Individual actions could sometimes be considered as eccentricity or temporary (having a 'turn' or 'going queer' were popular terms), but when the mental state of these men was displayed in public, especially when they turned violent, it was much more difficult to disguise or ignore. An example of a relatively simple episode is that of Private H, who had enlisted in October 1916 and served in France before being discharged in July 1919. He was wounded twice and also burnt by gas. In Australia he was first admitted to hospital for a mental condition in August 1921 and subsequently admitted to a Repatriation Hospital, diagnosed as 'disability shell shock? Mental'. His case notes reported that he had been admitted 'by ambulance due to shell shock—is a mental case.' He kept asking 'foolish questions' and had been 'violent on at least one occasion'. His father told asylum staff that his son had been 'queer' since his return from the front eighteen months previously. The Repatriation Commission recommended a war disability 'in view of patient's field service and medical report.'[37] There is no further information on this man and whether he made a full recovery or deteriorated remains a mystery. The father's use of the word 'queer', another folk diagnosis of the time, still hides the effect his son's condition had on his family and those around him.

Even before the war was over experts had recognised the likely potential for shell-shocked men to exhibit strange behaviours which might lead them to break the law. During the twenties the courts were no strangers to errant neurotics brought before them on all sorts of charges for anti-social behaviour from obscene language to murder. One author has gone so far as to conclude that in the early interwar years 'the diggers came to be regarded as "terrorists", "peculiar" and "mental"'.[38] These possibilities were recognised by sympathetic medical officers within the Repatriation Department. One wrote that it was 'quite reasonable to suppose that discharged men who have been for any length of time exposed to the strain and stress of battlefield conditions' might be unbalanced. He singled out 'those who have become neurasthenic resulting from shell shock and severe head injuries.' It was this type of patient who might 'during periods of recurring illness and often aggravated by environment, alcoholism and allied abuses—have recourse to the committal of crimes that in normal circumstances would be quite foreign to their temperament and disposition.'[39] The high incidence of this socially unacceptable behaviour contributed to this group's increasingly being sidelined by, then distanced from, conventional society and the way it wanted to remember the 'Great War'.

In all of this the public supporters of war neurotics could, at the same time, be seen both as a support to the state and a nuisance. These two views represent both ends of the spectrum and it is no accident that returned servicemen's associations feature in the two extremes. Service associations with their shared wartime experiences, not to mention financial resources and national network, were seen as logical, albeit informal extensions of state care. The Chairman of the Repatriation Commission wrote to the Prime Minister in July 1920 indicating one way in which these groups could help, particularly in keeping neurotic men out of the courts. He suggested that the Ex-Sailors and Soldiers Imperial League of Australia (ES & SILA) be approached and told that it would 'be performing a laudable service if it appointed officers to watch the interests of returned soldiers...when brought before the Courts and charged with civil offences.'[40] But the bottom line was that the Commission could see no reason for ex-soldiers to be treated differently under the law from anyone else.

Although well intentioned, the associations could actually negate professional efforts at healing shell-shocked ex-soldiers. The treatment and disposal of the military's mad was, according to Butler, based on 'the strange—though ethically arguable—premise insisted upon by the Returned Soldiers' Association—that the insane soldier should not be acknowledged to be insane (because of the stigma attaching to insanity) but should be treated without any certificate of insanity and apart from civil patients.'[41] This push from ex-servicemen for appropriate treatment of their colleagues very much mirrored what was happening in the UK and New Zealand at the same time.

The other view is represented by a particular recommendation proposed by the Executive Committee of the Returned Sailors and Soldiers Imperial League (NSW). In view of the number of recent cases of men having committed breaches of the peace, 'admittedly the outcome of mental derangement due directly or indirectly to active service affectations' it urged the government to set up a system which would see ex-soldiers who had satisfied judges that they were 'not wilful law breakers except through the effects on their brain of such active service' detained 'under competent and *sympathetic* medical administrators.' Tellingly, they also wanted these men to be released 'governed by the reports of the medical officers in charge of the case, such medical officers, where possible, to be *doctors who have seen service under fire* [emphasis added]...'[42]

This is typical of the pressure applied to all government departments that dealt with injured soldiers to have war veterans (i.e. doctors who had been at the front) on the appropriate confirming authorities or boards. There was a popular, and not unfounded, belief that civilian doctors who themselves had no idea of the battle conditions under which their patients had fought, could not therefore make a valid judgment of their subsequent state of mind or the effect a physical injury, such as an explosion, might mean for such men.

Despite the increasing incidence of petty and other crime committed by these men, the reasons behind their behaviour were always recognised. Listing the misdemeanours of mentally affected ex-servicemen, Professor W. Osborne of the University of Melbourne wrote in 1918 to the Secretary of the Defence Department with some prescience. He suggested that, unless such men were 'violent or dangerous' he did not think they should be placed in an asylum, but nor 'should they I think be allowed to do just as they please.' He advocated a 'firm and kind control' over them while they were 'taught to follow something useful.' While he acknowledged that there would be failures 'at least we can say we have tried to do our duty towards them. I do not think that in such cases it should be our endeavour to see how soon we can get them off the pay roll but how soon we can bring them back again to their normal state. Probably numbers have been discharged and we might have to collect them again...'[43] While this was still a paternalistic approach with overtones of discipline both individual and imposed, Osborne was keen to see these men return to a 'normal', and therefore productive place in society.

Nonetheless, after the war, neurosis was not always a successful defence in civil cases. Ex-serviceman B. H. Wright, a law student, was sentenced to twelve months' imprisonment with hard labour in Grafton Gaol late in 1919 following a charge of misconduct with another man. Wounded in 1917, Wright had been sent to England and was there for about four months. He returned to duty and was blown up and buried, and later gassed in March 1918. Wright spent time in several hospitals before returning to France where he was again blown up and evacuated to England. He returned to Australia in April 1919 at which time 'he complained of loss of memory.' He had also started to drink.[44] Other ex-soldiers were vulnerable in this sort of mental state. A leading psychologist was moved to write to a senior Defence bureaucrat citing his revulsion at both the vulnerability of, and the depths to which the shell-shocked serviceman had fallen. 'One case I have in mind is that of a shell shocked and discharged soldier who I was informed had got into the hands of a female harpy and this creature apparently for monetary gain was inducing the man to cohabit with her on a beach and his endeavours were revolting.' He described another case concerning 'a discharged soldier named O'Mara who robbed his mates in one of the [convalescent] homes and was arrested and charged with the theft...The judge discharged the man from trial without bringing him before a jury.'[45] Magistrates, many of them ex-officers, were still generally lenient in such cases.

Of course the mental state of some ex-servicemen could become too much—even for their spouses. This was especially the case where such men turned to physical abuse in the home. One Charlie Clifton went too far and one night attacked his wife and broke a bottle over her head. This proved one assault too many for Annie Clifton who 'drew a razor across his throat and killed him.' Her defence counsel stated that her husband had attacked her several times and a jury handed down a verdict of manslaughter.[46] Charlie, a Boer War veteran, had enlisted in the 34th Battalion in December 1915 but was almost immediately bundled off to the Parramatta Asylum. In 1917 he re-enlisted using old attestation papers and sailed for England. He got no closer to the front than Napsbury Hospital and was returned to Australia and, after a period of being absent without leave, was admitted to Broughton Hall before being released. Annie's is just one of many personal tragedies brought on by the psychological consequences of a horrible war.

The Repatriation Department—Help or Hindrance?

As we have seen, the matter of pensions and who or what administered them came to be an important one during the twenties, especially if the family was dependent on a pension for income. For some it became the focus of their life. Mr I was a 53-year-old ex-serviceman who was admitted to Callan Park with neurasthenia in January 1931. He had been shell shocked in Messines fifteen years earlier and had first become acquainted with the asylum system in 1923 when he was admitted to Randwick Hospital with depression before being discharged. He was initially refused a pension, but this was later granted some time before 1931. His case notes state that he talked about his pension '*ad nauseam*' and was obsessed with it.[47] Confusion about the war neurotic's entitlements to a pension continued apace.

On his return to Australia in 1919, J. W. Springthorpe was not impressed with what he found given his own recent experience of the satisfactory treatment of 'Soldier's Heart' in Britain at least as early as 1916 and its place in the War

Office pension calculations in 1918. He wrote to the Repatriation Commission on 14 July 1920 complaining that, on his return to Victoria in February 1919, he discovered that none of these developments had found their way to the southern hemisphere. 'Only last week the Caulfield Repatriation Sub-Committee sent me a man called Keene whose incapacity had been assessed at 1/3rd [disabled] when at a glance at the table approved and used by the War Office could have shown that it should have been estimated at 60%...Under present conditions such mistakes and unfairness are almost bound to occur in a large percentage of cases.'[48] The fact that he had been appointed as a part-time medical officer to the Repatriation Commission must have made his frustration all the worse. But if there was confusion in the minds of some, at least the Repatriation Commission was beginning to clarify what sorts of mental trauma it was dealing with.

According to its 1921 annual report, the Commission's experts had identified three classes of ex-soldiers who might be affected by war neuroses. The first and largest group included normally healthy men who 'develop a neurosis of an "anxiety" type, and become pure neurasthenics'. The second group comprised men whose 'family history is bad, and have always suffered from nervous disorders "neuropaths".' They could be expected to present with 'a rather hysterical symptom of some sort, such as paralysis, a contracture, aphonia, or stammering.' The Commission believed that these men would be 'exceedingly hard to treat, as the reflex effects of the injury are at times so great as to lead to organic changes, the true nature of which is not yet understood, further complicating the diagnosis and leading to a fixation of the symptoms which become practically ineradicable.' Curiously, the third group consisted of ex-soldiers 'whose development was deficient as regards their glandular structures'—men of a 'lymphatic type'. Apparently they would suffer from fatigue syndrome accompanied by general nervousness. Typically 'they had invariably seen little fighting and had not been vigorous workers as far as could be ascertained before the war.' This was as much a moral as a scientific observation.

This type of classification exudes middle-class condescension tinged with moral approbation. The Commission's experts believed that most of these neurosis cases developed after return from the war and after discharge, and they often found that there had been some added trigger in civil life 'such as marital infelicity, disappointments in marriage, over-indulgence in alcohol etc.' They failed to link causation between any of these and the neurosis itself. As for treatment, they admitted that hypnotism had 'proved exceedingly helpful in selected cases' and even psychoanalysis, although 'laborious work', could achieve success. But they concluded that the 'unintelligent man is a problem.' They did not know how to

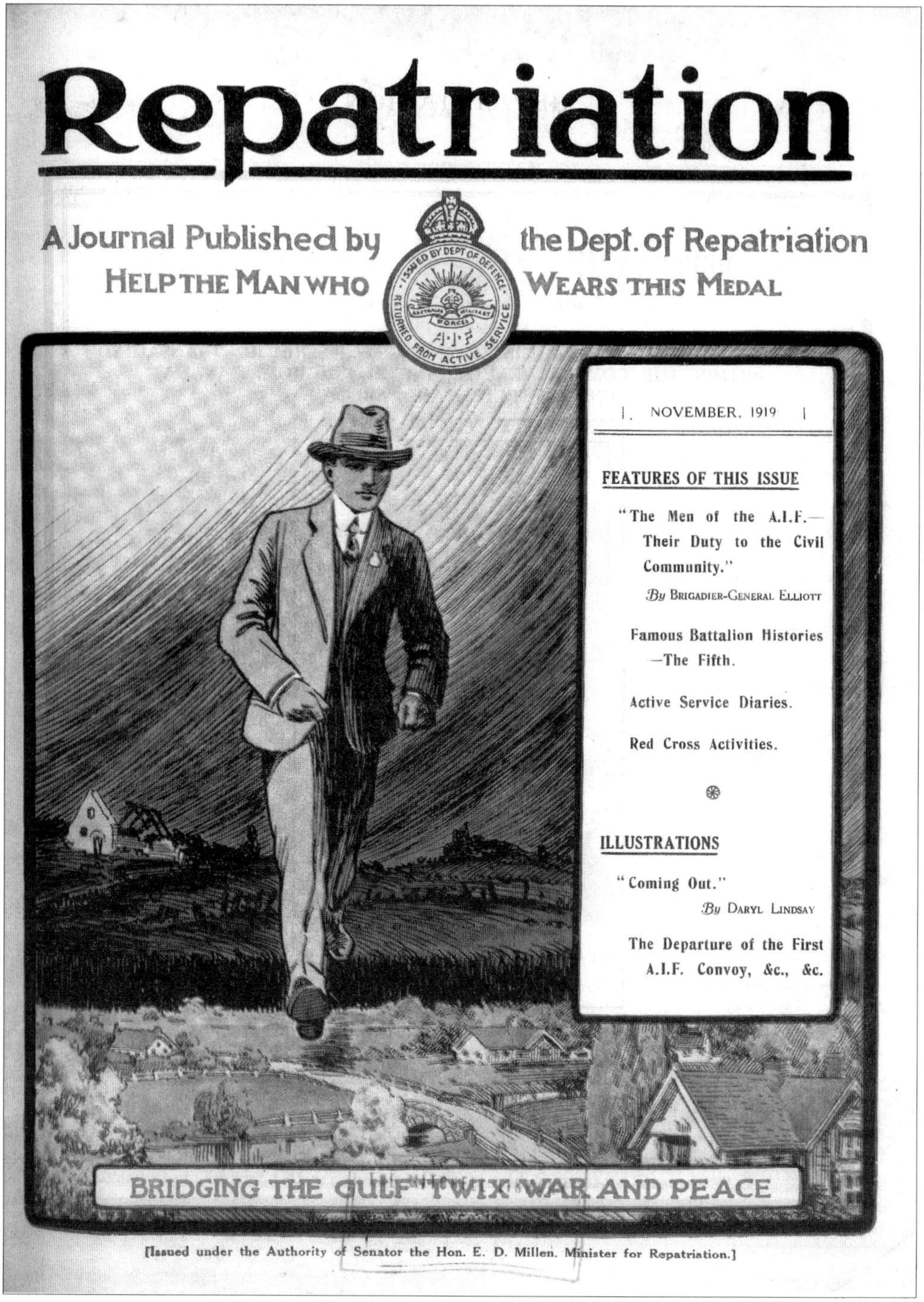

Cover of *Repatriation* magazine, 1 November 1919.
Despite its best efforts Australian repatriation authorities were not always successful in bridging the gap between reality and soldiers' expectations.

deal with him other than by 'sympathy and strong persuasion...' Neurasthenics were easier to treat, requiring only rest (but not prolonged), together with 'encouragement, short holidays, and light work.'[49] By the late 1930s the view which had evolved and that now pervaded repatriation circles was that, in mentally ill ex-servicemen 'the essential factor in their disablement is a constitutional psychopathic personality.'[50] Even so the Commission provided high quality medical treatment for servicemen through a system of repatriation hospitals and psychiatric cases were treated within this system.[51]

Some scholars argue that A. G. Butler, as well as Dr A. C. Courtnay and others in the Repatriation Department, 'believed in the transitory and environmental origin of the minor instances of shell-shock.' According to this theory, 'the only reasons for the number of postwar cases were either continuing stress in civilian life unrelated to war conditions, or the desire of some to remain ill in order to obtain compensation to which they were not entitled.'[52] This is probably too harsh on Butler, although his scepticism in this regard is easily understood from the many fraudulent claims he witnessed early in the war. Courtnay's biases however, are harder to fathom as it appears that he did not serve in the war. With a breathtaking assuredness he was still claiming as late as 1935 that 'war service had no lasting effect on the general health of soldiers.'[53] Billy Hughes, the Minister responsible for repatriation at the time felt moved to rebuff Courtnay publicly. But a number of senior bureaucrats would continue to share Courtnay's views for decades.

Fortunately, both for the men involved and for the Australian military, the Repatriation Commission clearly identified the inability of the latter to care for its own in the matter of psychological problems. In a 1924 agreement between Victoria and the Commonwealth, the Commission advised the Crown Solicitor that, as it was 'necessary to utilise the State machinery both statutory and other for the treatment of ex-soldiers patients it would be beneficial to the welfare of the patients to have them cared for by the Lunacy Department.'[54]

Peace or Peace of Mind?

In Britain 'servicemen who had suffered as a result of their wartime experiences soon faced a new threat: denial of their existence.'[55] While this was not the universal experience of shell-shocked ex-servicemen in Australia, some would continue to suffer, often at their own hands. Others were cared for in asylums or retained within the family circle. Of course vast numbers conquered their demons and led a 'normal' life as did others who had been successfully treated by psychologists. In reflective mood, and with another world war looming, Butler mirrored popularly held medical and social views in one of the most interesting paragraphs of his three-volume medical history of the war:

> The most important feature of so-called war neurosis...has been that for the most part it is not 'war' and is commonly not a 'neurosis' in the accepted medical sense, but is *a disability of conduct* [emphasis added] that comes more properly within the field of *morale*.[As for the various categories of neuroses] these were cured or became 'incurable', and in their place there appeared—especially in the years of the financial depression, 1930-1935, a manifestation of the same tendencies which, as we have seen, were at the root of acute 'shell shock'.[56]

To the extent that psychological weaknesses in men were denied in Australia, they hindered basic solutions to equally complex social needs—needs that were effectively cemented over in postwar years by Bean and others who influenced interwar Australian society. The interwar years would see isolated psychological successes, but a rise in the number of ex-service personnel with neuroses. With public reluctance to discuss shell shock and with the Treasury instigating stricter scrutiny of pensions as a result of a shift in priorities, the nation realised that it could not meet the promises made in the halcyon days after the war's end.

Endnotes

1 There are statistics for the state of Australia's early mental health. In Victoria in 1901 the rate of admissions to asylums for adult males aged between 25 and 30 was 12.77 per 10,000 of its population, while in New South Wales, for the age group 20–25 the rate was 8.05 per year. The source document provides no data for the 25–30 year range. W. Beattie-Smith and A.O. Powys, 'Insanity in Victoria and New South Wales', *Australasian Medical Gazette*, 20 June 1906, pages 660 and 662.

2 Shepherd, *A War of Nerves*, p. 151.

3 Winter, 'Shell-shock and the Cultural History of the Great War', p. 8.

4 Thompson, *Anzac Memories*, p. 151.

5 Ibid., p. 252.

6 *Singleton Argus*, 'Soldiers and Crime', 12 February 1920.

7 Gammage, *The Broken Years*, p. 270.

8 A resilient rump in the medical profession in the interwar period did not help them. 'Even sound [medical] teachers would deplore the use of the word "neurotic" as something to be passed over lightly and pointed out how important it was to try to discover an organic cause.' Allan Walker, *Clinical Problems of the War*, Australia War Memorial, Canberra, 1952. Volume I, Series 5 (Medical) *Australia in the War of 1939–1945*, pp. 674–5.

9 Damousi, *Freud*, p. 47.
10 Latham replied on 18 March 1935 to a request from Arthur Butler for more information on psychoses and neuroses. Personal Narratives, Captain Oliver Latham, No.1 AGH, AWM 41[1935].
11 See Jan Bassett, *Guns and Brooches*, Oxford University Press, Melbourne, 1992.
12 Butler, *Official History*, vol. III, p. 790.
13 Stone, 'Shellshock and the Psychiatrists', p. 167.
14 Based on figures in A. G. Butler, *Official History*, vol. III, p. 965.
15 Ibid., p.761.
16 Raftery, *Marks of War*, p. 22.
17 By 1930 pensions of unmarried ex-members of the AIF would be held and administered on their behalf by the Repatriation Commission. A portion of their pension was deducted to pay for their maintenance at mental hospitals. 'Unmarried Members Afflicted with Lunacy'. G.188, NAA (Sydney).
18 Letter from Mrs. K. Newsome, 21 May 1918, ref. her son Jack in Callan Park, to the Minister for Repatriation (Mr. Millen). National Archives Australia (Canberra) A.2487 B18/7061.
19 Memorandum 16 November 1916, from the Officer Commanding No. 13 AAH (Broughton Hall Correspondence), 14/8980. State Records of New South Wales.
20 Springthorpe, 'War Neuroses and Civil Practice', p. 283.
21 Thompson, *Anzac Memories*, pp. 150–1.
22 Butler, *Official History*, vol. III, p. 832.
23 Mosse, 'Shell-shock as social disease', p. 104.
24 See Michael Tyquin, *Sir Neville Howse: Australia's First Victoria Cross Winner*.
25 Lloyd and Rees, *The Last Shilling*, p. 237.
26 AAMC Hospitals in Australia—Special Hospitals, Mental—No. 24 AAH 'Stromness', Cottesloe, Western Australia. AWM 32 [64].
27 The relationship between the paper and the Repatriation Commission ebbed and flowed. In a letter of 8 August 1922 the acting Deputy Commissioner wrote to a colleague that 'for some reason, which I am unable to fathom, *Smith's Weekly*, has, of recent months ceased its tirade of abuse of the Commission.' He put this down to its editor-in-chief, Claude McCay, having retuned from abroad. A2487. 1922/9833. NAA (Canberra).
28 George Blaikie, *Remember Smith's Weekly?*, Rigby, Sydney, 1966, p. 157.
29 This paper was financed by Sir James Joynton Smith, a great champion of the Australian soldier who converted his Sydney mansion to a 40-bed hospital for war neurotics.
30 *The Argus*, 29 July 1924, p. 9.
31 Letter dated 11 May 1918 from the Victorian Inspector General of the Insane to the Medical Superintendent, Royal Park. 'Report of the Inspector of Hospitals for the Insane 1917'. AWM 253 AIF 498/1/693.
32 Details outlined in a memorandum from the Chairman of the Repatriation Department to the Prime Minister's secretary, 6 November 1920. File: A 458.Q356/19. NAA (Sydney).
33 Butler, *Official History*, vol. III, p. 966.
34 Sir Philip Gibbs was a former war journalist who took a highly emotive stance on what many regarded as the human toll of a futile war. See also Barham, *Forgotten Lunatics of the Great War*, p.414, *n*26.
35 AWM 41 [737].
36 Arthur H. Samuels, 'Invisible Wounds' in *Repatriation*, 25 June 1919, p. 18.
37 The Case of Private H. J. Humphreys. A 2487/1922/13913. NAA (Canberra).
38 Judith Allen, *Sex and Secrets: Crimes Involving Australian Women since 1880*, Oxford University Press, Melbourne, 1990, p. 130.
39 Minute from Dr J. F. Agnew, PDMO, Repatriation Department, 14 April 1920, p. 2. A. 2489/1/1920/1739. NAA (Canberra).
40 Letter from Chairman of the Repatriation Commission to the Prime Minister, 13 July 1920. A. 2489/1/1920/1739. NAA (Canberra).
41 Butler, *Official History*, vol. III, pp. 761–2.

42 Letter dated 24 February 1920 from the General Secretary of the Returned Sailors and Soldiers Imperial League (New South Wales) of Australia to the Prime Minister. National Archives Australia (Canberra) A. 2489/1/1920/1739.
43 Professor W. Osborne, Minute 'Shell Shock and War Strain', dated 30 August 1918, to the Secretary of the Defence Department. AWM 27 376/216.
44 Case Papers (Australian Military Forces) 1915–1920, File 14/8957. State Records of New South Wales.
45 Osborne Minute 'Shell Shock and War Strain' listing misdemeanours of mentally affected ex-servicemen. AWM 27 376/216.
46 Undated newspaper clipping in File 14/8959 (Case Papers). State Records of New South Wales.
47 File 14/8991. State Records of New South Wales.
48 Papers of Dr J.W. Springthorpe, Series 5, Wallet 2 of 5. AWM 2DRL/0701.
49 Extract from the Report of the Repatriation Commission for the Year ending 30 June 1921. AWM 41 [278].
50 Dr Parkinson quoted in Butler, *Official History*, vol. III, p. 835.
51 Lewis, *Managing Madness*, p. 40.
52 Garton, *The Cost of War: Australians Return*, p.171.
53 *Sydney Morning Herald*, 3 April 1935, p. 10.
54 'Agreement between the Repatriation Commission and Victoria re Mental Patients'. A3280 P7945. NAA (Canberra).
55 Bourke, *Dismembering the Male*, p. 121.
56 Butler, *Official History*, vol. III, p. 833.

Chapter Eight
The Interwar and an Invisible generation

We have seen how shell shock-affected soldiers were treated in a military-medical context. We look now at the evolving attitude of the wider Australian community to shell shock as well as at individual clinical experiences. This approach enables us to place the problem in the context of the 'no man's land' of Australian psychiatry between 1914 and 1925, a profession described by one practitioner then as 'the suckling science of psychiatry.'[1]

Like Britain and much of Europe there was, after the war 'an atmosphere of middle-class anxiety about unrest and disorder.'[2] In Australia this was manifest in the existence of right-wing groups (heavily subscribed by ex-soldiers) who waited in the wings to suppress any Bolshevik tendencies which might fester in the cities' slums. This reactionary aspect of the twenties occurred at the same time as sympathy for the war's psychological casualties moved increasingly to either embarrassed silence or antipathy. This development also coincided with the very period in which previously 'unaffected' soldiers now began belatedly to present with neuroses of various kinds. 'Not only had shellshock effectively blurred the distinction between the "neuroses" and "insanity" but many chronically "war-strained" ex-servicemen were, by the early 1920s, being transferred to asylums as in-patients.'[3] In describing this phenomenon in Britain between the wars, Peter Barham speculated that 'some [war] pensioners woke up belatedly to the recall of memories which had lain hidden for years; but it seems also likely that doctors, in caring for these patients and their families down the years, woke up belatedly to an awareness of the long fuse of traumatised memory that was still burning in many of these former service men of the Great War.'[4] This manifestation was reflected in Australia too. For some, usually both the victims and their families, it came as a shock; but to the more enlightened in the military and in the medical profession, it had long been a social time bomb.

Ben Shepherd in his *A War of Nerves* states that the real point about shell shock in the culture of the1920s was that it undermined men's authority, 'and with it the traditional roles of the sexes in the family: men, supposed to be strong, self-controlled, the providers to the household, were reduced to being weak, self pitying, dependent creatures. Women, hitherto the main sufferers from mental illness, now became carers. For both sexes that was hard to handle.'[5] Despite lurid details of murders and violence during the twenties in her study of females and crime, one of Judith Allen's central tenets cannot be ignored: 'Women's bodies and minds absorbed much of the shock, pain and craziness unleased by the war experience.'[6] But some females might have had a harder time than others. In the bush, women had shared the burdens of day-to-day work more intimately with their menfolk and often against greater odds and dangers (fire and flood) than their urban counterparts. This was particularly so in Australia's isolated farms and rural communities. The problem was magnified further on so-called 'soldier settlements' in country regions. 'Families found it difficult to cope with men who were used to years of rough living in the army. They also found it difficult to understand how and why their men had changed. Censored letters and news reports had done little to inform civilians about the experiences of the men at the front, and when the soldiers came home it was difficult for them to communicate the nature and effects of their experience.'[7]

The postwar medical literature from Britain was not heartening, with frequent reports citing patients with sexual impotence or irreconcilable marriage breakdowns. Many partners could scarcely recognise their long-time spouses after four years of separation. Women had become used to, and enjoyed, a measure of independence, the younger men had matured, while all of them were still coming to grips with their own memories of what they had seen or done during those war years. 'James' was a 35-year-old labourer who was admitted to Broughton Hall in April 1930 with 'Delusional Melancholia'.[8] He had enlisted in 1914 with the infantry and had been blown up in France in 1918 and hospitalised for two months before being discharged in August that year with a twelve-month disability pension. But twelve years later he was still 'depressed, bursts into tears easily...is superficial, reticent and evasive.'[9] Such individuals were not easy to live with and many such men remained single by choice or became itinerant workers 'humping their swag' around the countryside, always restless, never forgetting. Under the classification of 'disabilities' suffered by members of the AIF who were receiving service pensions as at 30 June 1940, neuroses, psychoneurosis and mental disorders were the third-largest category (745 males) after old age and 'vascular' disease.[10]

While there was a recognised inability in many ex-soldiers to articulate their fears and memories, too much has been made of their reluctance to discuss mental problems. Joy Damousi has written that it was 'unmasculine and socially unacceptable' for men to discuss their emotions.[11] This fits well with the C. E. W.

Bean mould. Peter Leese is another who argues that 'this shame has meant that very few have spoken about shell shock' in his view because it was driven by a fear 'of letting down comrades...'[12] Apart from the popularly held belief that *no* shell shocked soldier *ever* spoke about his nightmares, there is little evidence to support this view. Certainly by the 1920s war neurotics were constrained by the increasing influence of Bean's vision for Australia which argued for self-discipline and stoicism. But even bush folklore had allowed men to come to terms with their problems through social intercourse, if not with families, then with mates. The argument that they never did so is overstated.

The fact that source material for this often hidden domestic aspect of the shell shock problem is difficult to find is no doubt due to the embarrassment and sometimes the stigma or even shame, which still attached in some cases to neurotic soldiers. 'The effect of shell-shock on relations between the sexes is perhaps the most fascinating area of the subject and the most hidden, for in that reticent age, it was not thought proper to wash dirty linen in public.'[13] But sufficient material, especially in soldiers' letters and the newsletters of ex-servicemen's associations, exists for us to see that mental problems were discussed, albeit in the limited sphere of family circles or service clubs and not in the cosy format expected by some scholars. The club-like atmosphere of the many ex-servicemen's associations also provided a ready outlet for soldiers' grievances and emotional experiences.

What also made it hard for soldiers either recovering from psychological problems or just maintaining their mental balance, was that Australia did not have the same economic base as Britain, France or the United States. It was still a largely agrarian society, so that many men, especially the shell-shocked, for whom the virtues of employment and 'fresh air' were the mainstay of their treatment, tried to 'make a go of it' on the land. But the poor quality of soldier settlement lots, the isolation and the harsh environment, too often led to domestic disaster or suicide. As the Great Depression loomed, the urban environment also became a hostile one for the fragile ex-soldier. In the mid-twenties Dr W. E. Jones, the Inspector General of the Insane for Victoria, listed the principal causes of insanity among patients admitted in 1926. They were: 'domestic trouble, including loss of relatives and friends; adverse circumstances, including business anxieties and work and overwork, fright and nervous shock, intemperance and venereal disease.'[14] It was obvious that increasing economic uncertainty made it much harder for some to keep their heads.

Based on coroners' reports, one 1945 study found that, of 5,450 males who committed suicide in New South Wales from August 1914 to December 1937, 634 or 11.6% were returned soldiers.[15] These figures are for one state only. The same study showed the link with the financial depression of 1930–32 in that there were no fewer than 120 deliberate suicides of ex-soldiers during those years and, subsequent to 1930, the number of suicides tended to be above average. Noteworthy too is that of all the suicides in this period, eighteen were by men guilty of murder.

Some soldiers who had not fought with the AIF could also find themselves badly done by, through no other fault than that of poor legislation. Although this incident refers to an 'Imperial service man' (i.e. a British migrant whose war pension was paid by that government), his plight suggests that, although men like him could be missed, they were not simply ignored by 'the system'. In 1926 this ex-solder was admitted to Callan Park Asylum with 'neurasthenia'. He was advised that, during his time there, both his war pension and his allowances would be stopped. One of the nursing sisters on his ward took it upon herself to write to a local MP, himself an ex-serviceman. Not surprisingly the Repatriation Commission took a dim view of this direct approach especially because one of its officers regularly made weekly visits to this (and other) institutions to ensure that all military inmates were being properly administered. Dr C. D. Hogg, Inspector General of the Insane for New South Wales, wrote to the Commission stating that while 'suitable action had been taken as regards Nurse__', he sympathised with the British man and 'would be glad to know whether the Repatriation Commission could not take the matter up with the Imperial Authorities to obviate the differential treatment accorded the Imperial and Australian soldier.' He also raised strong objections to 'persons suffering from mental disorders being treated any differently to persons suffering from any other form of disability arising from war service.'[16] It seems that some progress was being made at last in the official view of the shell-shocked soldier—at least in this part of Australia.

In Australia the diagnostic label of 'neurasthenia' remained in use through this decade, but only after it had changed from a physical into a psychic classification. It was during this period that the terminology of 'nerves' was replaced 'by the language of neuroses and psycho-neuroses, neurasthenia being reduced to just one psycho-neurotic symptom, namely abnormal fatigue.'[17] Neurasthenia continued to dominate ex-servicemen's postwar morbidity. 'Joseph', for example, was married, a wagon builder and 38 years old when admitted to Broughton Hall late in December 1925 with this particular condition. He was discharged only days later, his report noting simply that he had 'recovered' but giving no indication as to his treatment.[18] While deployed in France, a bomb had dropped near him from a German aeroplane and had destroyed a lorry he was repairing. His immediate response was to become very frightened and to run about crying. Before this he had never taken much notice of bombs, but afterwards, whenever his unit was bombed 'Joseph' would become so nervous that he had to leave the tent and run around looking for a hole in which to hide. Six years after the war he still could not sleep properly and, when he did fall asleep, he always woke in fright. He suffered constant pains in the head and had become absent-minded.[19]

Distressing though 'Joseph's' symptoms were, he was not teetering on the brink as were those who went on to develop psychoses. Some psychiatrists at the time who had seen front-line service themselves, such as the American practitioner Norman Fenton, were now classifying their patients into distinct psychiatric categories. Fenton had actually conducted a survey of almost eight hundred soldiers at the end of the war and had subsequently developed various categories of neuroses. These included the 'psychotic'—men who suffered both chronic and acute conditions including 'psychopathic personality', epilepsies and 'dementia praecox' (schizophrenia) and who required constant supervision and institutional care. There were 'fatigued' men who were able to work where jobs were available, 'but were unable to do so without personal discomfort and probable relapse.' Then came the 'neurotic' ex-servicemen 'who had full employment or were capable of full employment, but continually suffered from severe nervous difficulties and saw doctors either regularly or frequently.'[20] This classification is interesting as there is no comparable study of the AIF and, as mentioned, any data on which a study could be based has been largely destroyed. Although most American soldiers were not deployed to the Western Front for sustained periods, one suspects that there are valid comparisons with Australian soldiers.

Often it was left to wives or families to help doctors fill in the gaps in their patients' dossiers. Their story is the stuff of a separate book, for it was to the woman, often the wife or mother, but not infrequently sisters, sweethearts and also fathers, that the burden of years of care fell. Some men were nursed or cared for at home until age, illness or violence caught up with them or their partner, after which they were committed to the state asylum system. It was the folk at home who were able to provide a 'before and after' portrait of their loved ones for doctors struggling to treat the war neurotic.

'Dennis' was single, 32, and a plasterer who was admitted to Broughton Hall for seven months in 1927. He had complained of headaches for the previous five years and his mother wrote this letter to the medical superintendent at Broughton Hall: 'I can only say that my son has complained of his head [sic] ever since he returned from France...Prior to the war he was quiet, easy going and easily satisfied...He was under arms from 11 August 1914...Since his return he has been irritable and argumentative.'[21] This man had served in New Guinea and France and, while not wounded or shell-shocked, he succumbed to trench fever in 1916 and was away from the front for six months. According to his clinical notes, he 'was in a nervous condition.' His situation illustrates that it was not just soldiers with front-line service who were liable to psychological problems as a result of their military service.

'Dennis' had also been treated 'by many medical men without apparent relief.' The reference to his seeking treatment from a number of doctors was not untypical of the period and reflects the ongoing uncertainty about definitive care. An unsigned letter from a returned soldier dated 6 March 1919 and addressed to Dr J. W. Springthorpe was found in the latter's files and clearly illustrates this: 'Sir, I have read in one of the newspapers of your marked success with soldiers suffering from nerve complaints. I have had "neuritis"—more or less severe—for over two years and I have been wondering whether you could do me any good.' He had seen four doctors, three specialists and been to a sanatorium three times. 'The Sanatorium squirted me with scalding water, ice water, electrified water and salt water, also treated me to some electric light baths, sulphur baths, enema injections and massage every day. After two years I can say truthfully that not one of them ever did me the least benefit...'[22] Other cases were not what they seemed.

'Edward's' sister was instrumental in providing medical authorities with a history of her brother's unusual behaviour. 'Edward' was admitted to Broughton Hall in 1925 with 'paraphrenia'. He was 29, single and worked as a clerk. He had spent six months in Egypt and France before being invalided home for shell shock. According to his medical file however, while he 'was in a nervous state...it is not true that he was blown up, as he told the authorities. He really became too funked [scared] to face things, nerves gave way and to make his case look genuine he told a lie about his being blown up. Admits it was uncourageous but he was built that way and couldn't help it.' 'Edward' then started drinking heavily twelve months after he returned to Australia. 'He was nervous of people in authority, [experienced] lack of concentration and hypochondria.' His sister wrote that, since his return in 1917, he had been 'strange in his manner. He seemed to be indifferent to all around him, and he has been most reticent the whole time. At home he rarely spoke...he always appeared in a dazed condition...'[23] Was he living out his own phantom shell shock?

Those who have interviewed old soldiers note 'the awkwardness and pain of the domestic no man's land between army and civilian life.' There were bound to be wider repercussions. 'The national divorce rate doubled between the censuses of 1911 and 1921 and women brought the majority of the petitions for divorce for the first time.'[24] It is not hard to see why. Letters from the often silent, long-suffering but loving, partners of war neurotics flesh out what had happened in ordinary families after the war.

'Bill' was a 38-year-old married miner who, during the war, had been gassed and wounded. 'Bill' was admitted to Broughton Hall in August 1925 for a week with 'paraphrenia' and his wife wrote a letter to the medical superintendent with 'Bill's' history:

> Dear Sir, In regards to my husband's sickness I can only attribute it to the strenuous times he had during the war...He never seems to be able to get a night's sleep and has often complained of headaches...He has been doctoring himself for the last two years but has only got worse, couldn't get him interested in anything and he wouldn't go out anywhere, would say he was trying to get better in his own way.

On the last day at Broughton Hall he twice assaulted a night attendant. His clinical notes stated that 'Bill' had 'never been the same since returning from the war. Any little noise makes him jump. Likes to be in company, as this helps him from being despondent. He has not the same confidence in himself as formerly.'[25] The reference to company is important, for this was one material aid that clubs and ex-servicemen's associations could offer these men. Deplored by wowsers and many dutiful wives alike for their boozy activities, they nonetheless acted as a sounding board for memories either shared or understood by comrades. One servicemen's paper, *The Rising Sun*, defended their role: 'Why the [R.S.&S.] Club Movement? [Clubs] made better men and helped many unfortunate diggers to get out of that recluse mind and the reaction of war service that most of us have or still suffer from...'[26] These same groups often raised funds to support widowed women, helped to find work for or provided character witnesses at court appearances for men whose mental condition had affected their behaviour.

The cases of three other individuals illustrate not only the complexity of their own neuroses but the probable consequences for family and friends and why so few war neurotics could hold down steady jobs. The first case is that of 'John', who was admitted to Broughton Hall in 1924 with 'chronic alcoholism' and discharged a few days later—presumably after 'drying out'. Aged 36, he was still single and had been a grazier. He enlisted in August 1914 and was subsequently wounded and shell shocked in August 1915 at Lone Pine and was repatriated to Australia in December. He sold his 5,000-acre property due to a very poor season and, by 1923, he was drinking a bottle of whisky a day, despite never having drunk alcohol prior to Gallipoli. 'Has disturbing dreams, eats badly, sleeps badly, generalised tremor of whole body when excited.'[27] 'Harold' is the second case, and was a 36-year-old veterinary surgeon admitted to an asylum with 'depression' in July 1924 and discharged 'recovered' the following month. He had enlisted as a signaller in 1915 and was buried alive at Gallipoli and 'sustained nervous debility and melancholia. He remained well until 1921 when he began to suffer from insomnia. He collapsed in November 1923, recovered and collapsed again in February 1924. He became very depressed, hysterical (uncontrolled excitement), shaky.'[28]

Finally, there is the story of a former officer whose mental state was the subject of a clinical paper by Dr Idris Morgan, who proclaimed the efficacy of hypnotic suggestion as a cure for shell shock. 'Fred' had been both wounded and concussed in a raid in France in 1916. Subsequently he suffered amnesia concerning the event as well as developing paralysis of the right arm. He returned to Australia where 'isolation, explanation, electricity and massage had been used in treatment. Scars upon the arm bear evidence of the application of a cautery [a hot iron for surgical sealing]. An attempt had been made to induce hypnosis in a military hospital, but as it had been made in a ward without a screen it had been unsuccessful.'[29] When Morgan saw this patient the man was suffering from uncontrolled fits of rage, pain in his arm and neck, regular lapses of memory, frequent terrifying nightmares and depression and he could not work. In 1923 Morgan subjected the man to four successive 'sittings' of hypnosis and claimed his patient was symptom-free. His patient had a relapse some weeks later due to pressures of business, but Morgan again intervened and claimed there had been 'no recurrence of any symptoms in the following three years.'[30]

Some men elicited profoundly different attitudes as a result of their war experience. This case, involving an ex-artilleryman in 1918, is not untypical and, for those who survived, it was this type of neurotic who lived out of the public view in various 'Repat' or other institutions. Gunner 'Jack' was a former deep-sea diver and therefore used to danger. He was admitted to Broughton Hall at the end of the war in a sad state. He had been 'wounded at Passchendaele Ridge with 50 pieces of shell taken out, two teeth knocked down his throat, two wounds to back of head, one eye knocked out, the other taken out three days later, left arm and hand partially paralysed, several wounds under left shoulder and one under heart.' On his return to Sydney he had also walked off the wharf at Circular Quay and was presumably rescued. In 1920 the medical superintendent of Broughton Hall was not happy to take him back again 'because he is extremely difficult to control and, being blind, he has the sympathy of so many people...If he came back I expect that it would be necessary to certify him as he would no doubt decline to conform to the regulations of the hospital. He appears now to be mentally bad and suffers from delusions of persecution and hallucinations of hearing. He has friends in Sydney and I am afraid that their misplaced sympathy and interference would render his care very difficult. I suppose it would not be possible to prevent his return to New South Wales, but could he not be cared for in Western Australia until he can be declared mentally well and free from his delusions?'[31] The moral tone in this letter is barely disguised. 'Jack' was drinking heavily by this time. Was it from shame or frustration? As Peter Leese so eloquently phrased it 'some combatants were irrevocably shattered by the war, they suffered guilt and shame in silence, they were either too little or too much aware of their own traumatic neurosis.'[32]

Outside the home there was sometimes a fear or mistrust of the neurotic soldier and the most obvious expression of this attitude was employers' reluctance to hire anyone deemed to be 'queer'. This denied these men the means of attaining the very cure that medical professionals sought for their patients' long-term recovery from self-doubt or neuroses. 'According to many veterans, the very name of their condition was enough to put off employers, and if the man in question had visible signs of mental disturbance, a bad stutter or a functionally paralysed hand, the stigma was greater and the chance of making a good impression even more remote.'[33] Ex-service organisations railed against such prejudice but it continued into the 1930s.

The grim realities of the economic malaise in the late twenties also made an impact on the treatment of neurotic soldiers. In 1928 the acting Premier of New South Wales summoned a cabinet meeting to consider the steps to be taken to improve conditions at the state mental hospitals. He said that a substantial increase in the estimates would be necessary to raise standards in these hospitals to an acceptable level. 'He had visited several of the institutions and found the conditions heartbreaking.'[34] The situation was no better in Victoria, home of the second-largest mental health establishment in Australia. There, the state's Inspector General, Dr W. E. Jones, noted in his annual report for 1928 that more accommodation was required to meet growing demand. Apart from the 5,552 persons (almost evenly balanced between the sexes) registered as insane in that state, there were 134 patients who were in military mental hospitals and a further 35 ex-servicemen who were out on 'leave of absence.'[35] By the mid-thirties, with increasing economic uncertainty, there had been little improvement. In 1935 the New South Wales Inspector General of Mental Hospitals repeatedly drew attention 'to the totally inadequate provision made for his department and to the impossibility of giving his patients the treatment that they should have.'[36]

After the war, the Repatriation Department took over the military hospital system and its mental hospitals. Each state had an elaborately equipped repatriation hospital in its capital city and the Australian Red Cross Society continued to liaise with these institutions through the provision of official visitors, amusements such as cinemas and additional recreational and therapeutic equipment. Military institutions were generally better off because of greater public scrutiny, the system of official visitors and the continued support of the Red Cross. *The Argus* reported on the 1930 Returned Sailors and Soldiers Conference. It had moved a resolution requesting 'that the Federal Government make available a compassionate allowance now at its disposal or provide another special fund for cases where former soldiers and their dependants are in distressed circumstances, as result of such former soldiers developing mental trouble or diseases where there is a possibility of these diseases being due to war service.'[37]

There were still differences in standards in asylum accommodation between the states, with the smaller states often being in a better position because there were fewer patients in their institutions. For example, in the early 1920s, South Australia's Parkside was caring for only fourteen soldiers before they were moved in 1929 to Norfield where a much larger and purpose–built mental hospital had just been completed. The new hospital boasted a special repatriation block. New South Wales and Victoria, however, were regularly berated by the press for the overcrowded state of their hospitals (and had been since the turn of the century). In fact there was a sensation in Victoria in 1921 when rumours spread of the forcible transfer of ex-soldier patients from No.16 AAH (Mont Park) to state asylums at Kew and Sunbury.[38] After much waving of paper in both the commonwealth and state parliaments, it transpired that these men were being moved to alleviate temporary overcrowding pending the completion of new accommodation for them.

By 1930 accommodation shortages for the mentally ill were becoming acute. In that year Victoria's premier estimated that there was a shortage of 450 beds, despite an earlier agreement with the Repatriation Department that it would expand military accommodation at Bundoora. He stated that there were more than 136 ex-soldiers in asylums around his state.[39] However this decade was not the static backwater that has often been depicted. In 1934 the Repatriation Commission paid for new buildings at Callan Park to accommodate one hundred mental patients, while in 1935 it repealed earlier legislation and consolidated its mental health legislation, as did the government of South Australia in the same year.[40] Even so, ex-military patients continued to fare relatively better than their civilian counterparts, even in the same institutions.

"ONE OF THE WHITEST"

"Paddy" Hauenstein's Fate

DIGGER MATES AT FUNERAL

"Poor old Paddy! He was one of the whitest; but he never got a fair go!"

This remark was voiced by one of the many digger comrades of Dennis Hauenstein, who followed his hearse to

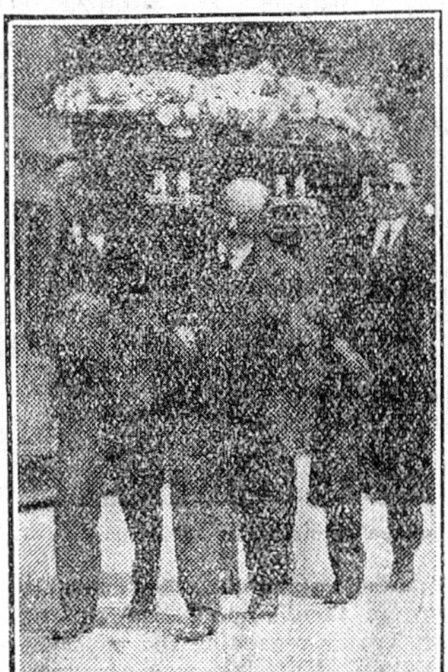

ON THE WAY TO ROOKWOOD
The remains of Dennis Hauenstein on the Sydney mortuary station this afternoon.

the graveside at Rookwood this afternoon.

Hauenstein returned from five years' service at the front in 1919, with a fine record and the rank of lieutenant, gained on the field. To conform with tradition, he should then have settled down to a quiet and comfortable life; but instead he was dogged by misfortune to the day of his tragic death.

Out of work and desperate for money to support his wife and young family, his continuous ill-luck culminated in his pitiful attempt to rob the Hurlstone bank, and his subsequent suicide by poisoning.

There was a pathetic scene in Wood Coffill's George-street mortuary when Mrs. Hauenstein, with her eldest daughter, aged 13, visited the chapel to see the face of her husband for the last time.

When the lid of the coffin was lifted, she reeled, and would have fallen had not someone caught her. Sobbing bitterly, she was led back to her seat.

Besides Mrs. Hauenstein and her daughter, the mourners included the father of the deceased, Mr. H. Hauenstein; two sisters, Mrs. Wheeler, and Miss Ettie Hauenstein; and a brother, Mr. William Hauenstein.

It was during this decade that the Repatriation Commission took on the mantle of ogre in the popular mind and, in this regard, it has often been reviled in the decades since. But it did go to extraordinary lengths in the case of mentally ill ex-soldiers to ensure that their claims, where justified, were acted upon and suitable pension entitlements paid. By the 1930s the Commission continued to be sensitive to what it saw as negative and unfair criticism and hostility by the ex-servicemen's lobby to its treatment of mentally ill soldiers. This newspaper item was typical of many at the time.

Concerned at the implication that there was an increased incidence of insanity amongst those who served during the war, the Commissioner ordered an inquiry. In his response to the inquiry, the Senior Medical Officer (NSW) stated that he believed 'the incidence of insanity in ex-soldiers is very much similar to that in the general male population of similar age' although he admitted that the 'lack of precise statistics in the matter is regrettable.'[41] Subsequently he ordered a search of mental asylums in New South Wales and found that there were 450 ex-soldiers among their certified inmates. He asserted that there was a ratio of 1:200 ex-military personnel certified in 1934–35 in comparison with the civilian ratio of 1:155 in the comparable male population.

With the passing of the years a sort of social amnesia settled on Australia. Despite the solemnity of the pledge 'Lest We Forget' at various state commemorative ceremonies every year, the neurotic soldier began to fade from public sight and consciousness—not least within the military. 'It is noteworthy, even in the records of war pensions in asylums, how rarely from about the mid-1920s onwards the war is remarked upon, as though even the mentally disturbed had decided to leave their memories of the war behind and to go about their daily business as mental patients, only uttering the sorts of preoccupations and complaints that mental patients were supposed to utter.'[42] Bean's sanitised ideal of the nation state was now complete. It was just as well his vision excluded the mentally war-damaged. Dane reported in 1926 that he had subjected twelve war neurotics 'to complete analysis' and contended that 'the underlying basis was a disturbance of the infantile sexual *libido*, the outstanding factors being either a strongly developed homosexual component or a high degree of narcissism.'[43] This was a view that would have not endeared him to the military establishment, nor did it fit Bean's idea of an exclusively heterosexual (i.e. 'normal') society. But to the strongly heterosexual ex-servicemen's associations who had by now become embarrassed at reminders of their members' brief flirtation with sensitivity and tenderness to distressed comrades in the trenches, it was anathema.

The Evolution of Psychiatry in Australia

Between the wars Australia took its lead from Britain in matters concerning the management of its military casualties and the administration of its mental health infrastructure. Anything new was picked up quickly and, where possible, assimilated or picked over for local application. For example, in October 1928, all state Repatriation Commissioners were circularised with a recently released report from the British Deputy Commissioner of Pensions pointing out the relevance of the report 'in respect to the problems encountered in Australia re accommodation, occupations, segregation etc.'[44] Under this umbrella, home-grown developments continued apace.

Freud was finally acknowledged in Australia for his contribution to psychoanalysis, and the unconscious mind 'which psychologists once asserted to be non-existent, has become the most important department of psychology.'[45] Paul Dane, by this time one of the leading lights in Australia, was characteristically blunt in his assessment of the postwar period. Writing in a medical journal he noted that 'the problem of the genesis and treatment of the psycho-neurotic soldier is still one that remains to be solved.' He went on to explain the plethora of diagnostic and other terms then in use. The list of conditions which led to admission throughout the 1920s included: melancholia, dementia praecox, psychosis, neurosis, dipsomania, paraphrenia, congenital mental deficiency, manic depression, hysteria, exhaustion. By the 1930s doctors were still using DAH as a diagnostic label.

Dane wrote that in 'very few cases are the signs and symptoms so well defined as to enable a definite clinical label to be attached' and he used classifications such as anxiety states, compulsion neurosis, conversion hysteria and organic conditions with which a psycho-neurotic disturbance is associated.[46] The situation was little better in the field of legislation. Despite progress throughout the interwar years there was little movement towards uniform lunacy laws. This was the plea of W. Ernest Jones to a medical gathering in March 1934 in which he also argued for 'reciprocity between the States in dealing with the treatment of mental deficiency and the interstate recognition of medical certificates.'[47]

Between the wars there was no Commonwealth legislation comparable to Britain's *Mental Treatment Act 1930*, with most of the states clinging to their own acts. However in 1936 the Commonwealth Government introduced a system of service pensions under which ex-servicemen and women could obtain old age benefits at 'an age and under conditions more favourable than the rest of the community.'[48] While there was no specific provision for mental disability, one of the grounds for claiming a pension was permanent unemployability. The war and its psychological casualties were now recognised and the place of psychology in the broader medical establishment was assured. In Sydney a new Associate Chair of Psychology was established in 1921 and the University of Hobart created a chair in 1922. Elsewhere other courses, abandoned during the war, were reconstituted in Melbourne, Perth and Brisbane.[49]

Outside academia there were few practising psychiatrists. A former member of the Australian Army Medical Corps and a Military Cross amputee, Dr Roy Winn was Australia's first full-time practising and *trained* psychiatrist. He began to exert a professional and certainly more positive approach to the war neurotic. The wider medical profession began to realise, belatedly perhaps, the place of psychiatry in the effective treatment of war neurosis. In reviewing F. C. Bartlett's newly published *Psychology and the Soldier* in England in 1928, Dr Morris Miller could still applaud Bartlett's plea that 'the military authorities should provide adequate facilities for psychological research'—a plea 'that should have been made in Australia in the interests of repatriation.'[50]

The profession was still checked by the belief, held by a number of eminent practitioners, in the link between hereditary predisposition and soldiers' mental problems. Their thinking may have been influenced by the popularity of the eugenics movement in Australia between the wars—a development that seemed to sit well with the increasing nationalism and a contemporary trend to right wing politics. Australian medical doctors such as Professor R. J. Berry and Dr Oliver Latham subscribed to the hereditary theory, but serious mental deficiency 'only accounted for some of the problem...There were some men who were "naturally" nervous, and it was this type of soldier who succumbed to the stress of war. This was an approach supported in large measure by many psychiatrists and doctors.'[51] In a letter to the *Medical Journal of Australia* in 1935, Arthur Butler asked 'for guidance', as he believed that it was 'a matter that deeply concerns the public weal both in peace and war.'[52] He seems then to have begun to query the part heredity played in mental disorders, opting now for environmental and nurturing factors as disposing factors to shell shock and other psychoses.

In reflecting on the war, Arthur Butler determined that only 906 recruits had been rejected for 'psychoneuroses' as distinct from shell shock. A further 4,296 soldiers who had seen active service were repatriated with the same condition, while 290 others who had not been at the front were also returned to Australia—all diagnosed with psychoneuroses. Most of these men were entitled to pensions. Under the classification of 'organised mental diseases', the military rejected 925 recruits, while 589 men who had served at the front returned to Australia together with another 261 soldiers who had never fired a shot. Sixty-five recruits were rejected for 'moral defects' (unspecified, but presumably including venereal disease and alcoholism), 99 front-line soldiers and 20 others were sent home for the same reason.[53]

In 1921 the Repatriation Commission confidently asserted that nervous diseases due to war service had ceased to be 'a prominent feature in hospitals and the streets.' The reference here to 'streets', and what therefore must have been the very public manifestation of military madness is significant. Within a few years this assessment seemed optimistic. Repatriation authorities were alarmed by the increase in successful applications for pensions arising from neurosis.[54] But, as we have seen, psychological issues continued to simmer away during the interwar years and, between 1936 and 1941, i.e. *after* the worst of the country's financial depression, there was a significant increase in the number of service pensions being paid to men for 'neurosis, psychoneurosis and mental disorders'—from 79 ex-servicemen in 1936 to 745 men in 1940.[55] The Repatriation Department treated 316 'mental patients' in 1922; 579 in 1932; and 520 ex-servicemen in 1941. However, despite their declining numbers, the total number of ex-servicemen treated for 'war neuroses' by the repatriation hospital system (including out-patients) rose from 1,570 in 1926 to 4,891 by 1939.[56]

Taking the months of May in a random sample from all military patients admitted to the Repatriation General Hospital in Caulfield over an eight-year period from 1926 to 1934, or an average of 157 admissions a month, only 5.5 were definitely identified as 'neurasthenia'. This represented a mental admission rate of about 30 per year.[57]

These figures still seem small and they may point to either a lingering lack of confidence in the system by ex-soldiers and their families (who therefore stayed away from these institutions), or to under-reporting. While there is a dearth of statistical data with which to make meaningful comparisons or draw conclusions, there is a small sample available from the New South Wales asylum system, obtained from ten such institutions from around that state in 1936.[58] There were 10,103 men (presumably these included out-patients, not just certified patients in long-term accommodation) in receipt of a Repatriation Department pension. Their average age was 47.2 years, but the figures include 176 ex-soldiers and sailors from Great Britain, New Zealand, Canada, South Africa and the United States. Of the 179 remaining men in this report whose war service could be unambiguously traced, 68 former infantrymen naturally formed the largest group, followed by the artillery, the Light Horse and pioneers, Medical Corps and so on down to one engineer. Despite their low numbers, the pioneers, those who laid mines, built tunnels bridges etc., and who were therefore sometimes in very dangerous situations, would appear to be over-represented for their relatively small numbers. Although statistically unsustainable, some very general comparisons may be made with the larger AIF.

Using the Commonwealth Government *Hansard* for 1 November 1935, we know the number of persons who served overseas with the 1st AIF totalled 331,781. These were classified by corps or employment as:

Flying Corps	2,275
Light Horse & Camel Corps	30,365
Artillery	25,105
Engineers, Signals	10,384
Infantry	210,981
Machine Gun Corps	4,476
Pioneers	3,970
Army Service Corps	9,735
Army Medical Corps	12,945
Other Details	21,545

The high incidence of some groups over others (taking into account the much larger numbers in infantry, for example, over other corps) reflects much of the anecdotal and direct evidence reviewed in earlier chapters.

In 1933 Cyril Burt, a British psychologist, delivered a lecture at the London School of Hygiene and Tropical Medicine. He declared that, more than any other agency, the Great War had 'brought home to the medical world the artificiality of the distinction between the normal mind on the one hand, and its abnormal condition on the other.'[59] But surprisingly quickly, the lessons learned not only by military medicine, but by Australia's military authorities and, more importantly in the longer term by repatriation officialdom, were forgotten or contested in the 'sure' knowledge of the advance of science between 1920 and 1940.[60]

Endnotes

1 R.S. Ellery, *The Cow Jumped Over the Moon: Private Papers of a Psychiatrist*, F. W. Cheshire, Melbourne, 1956, p. 88.

2 Eric Dean, 'War and Psychiatry: examining the diffusion theory in light of the insanity defence in post-World War I Britain', *History of Psychiatry*, vol. IV, 1993, p. 65. This should be read in conjunction with Allen's *Sex and Secrets: Crimes Involving Australian Women since 1880*. She describes some of the legal defences used by ex-soldiers in various crimes.

3 Stone, 'Shellshock and the Psychiatrists', p. 245.

4 Barham, *Forgotten Lunatics of the Great War*, p. 354.

5 Shepherd, *A War of Nerves*, p. 149.

6 Allen, *Sex and Secrets*, p. 131.

7 Thompson, *Anzac Memories*, p.152.

8 Broughton Hall and its patient 'mix' was not untypical of the other 'military' asylums around Australia at this time.

9 File: 14/8990. State Records of New South Wales.

10 Butler, *Official History*, vol. III, p. 967.

11 Damousi, *Freud in the Antipodes*, p. 39.

12 Leese, *Shell Shock*, p. 33.

13 Shepherd, *A War of Nerves: Soldiers and Psychiatrists*, p. 145. But it was not dealt with in John McQuilton's *Rural Australia and the Great War* (2001).

14 The Melbourne *Argus*, 7 December 1927, p. 20.

15 S. J. Minogue, 'Suicides Amongst returned Soldiers of the 1914-1918 War' in *MJA*, 24 February 1945, p. 195.

16 Letter, 24 November 1926. SP 948 G900 Part 1. NAA (Sydney).

17 M. Gijswijt-Hofstra and R. Porter (eds.), *Cultures of Neurasthenia from Beard to the First World War*, Amsterdam, 2001, p. 6.

18 In 1926 Dr Evan Jones reported that Australian mental hospitals had recovery rates (from all causes) of between 25 and 50 per cent. He gave his own institution's rate for 1925 as 50 per cent, while a further 20 per cent had been discharged 'improved.' 'Experiences in the Treatment of Voluntary Patients at the Psychiatric Clinic, Broughton Hall', *MJA*, 4 September 1926, p. 316.

19 File No: 14/8983. State Records of New South Wales.

20 Leese, *Shell Shock*, p. 135.

21 Letter dated 3 February 1927, File: 14/8983. State Records of New South Wales.

22 Unsigned letter to Springthorpe, Sydney, 6 March 1919 from a returned soldier. Papers of Dr J. W. Springthorpe, Series 5, Wallet 6 of 7. AWM 2 DRL/0701.
23 File No: 14/8983. State Records of New South Wales.
24 Thompson, *Anzac Memories*, p. 153.
25 File: 14/8983. State Records of New South Wales.
26 *The Rising Sun*, no. 2, vol. 1, editorial, December 1928.
27 File No: 14/8983. State Records of New South Wales.
28 Ibid.
29 Idris Morgan, 'Hypnotic Suggestion', *MJA*, 15 January 1927, p. 87.
30 Ibid.
31 Case Papers (Australian Military Forces) 1915–1920. File: 14/8957. State Records of New South Wales.
32 Leese, *Shell Shock*, p. 133.
33 Ibid., p. 153.
34 *The Argus*, 20 January 1928, p. 16.
35 *The Argus*, 28 November 1928, p. 9. By late 1930 these numbers had grown to 39 men in 'military wards' and 193 ex-servicemen classified as 'mental cases'. *The Argus*, 2 October 1930.
36 Editorial: 'The Mental Hospitals of New South Wales', *MJA*, 27 April 1935, p. 529. It has also been said that, from 1915 to 1940, 'Australia drifted into a backwater of social policy.' T. Carney and P. Hanks, *Social Security in Australia*, Oxford University Press, Melbourne, 1994, p. 33.
37 *The Argus*, 13 November 1930, p. 19.
38 See File: A458 745/1/339. NAA (Canberra).
39 Letter from the Premier to the acting Prime Minister, 19 September 1920. A.458 K368/5. NAA (Canberra).
40 Callan Park Mental Hospital, G394/1/4, NAA (Canberra).
41 Letter of 5 January1937, Senior Medical Officer to the Deputy Commissioner of the Repatriation Commission. SP 948/1 G530. NAA (Sydney).
42 Barham, *Forgotten Lunatics of the Great War*, p. 353.
43 Dane, 'Psychoanalysis and Psychotherapy' in *MJA*, December 1926, p. 853.
44 SP 948/1 G826. NAA (Sydney).
45 Roy Coupland Winn, 'Psychoanalysis and General Practice', *MJA*, 29 February 1936, p. 293.
46 Dane, 'The Psycho-Neuroses of Soldiers and Their Treatment', p. 427.
47 *Sydney Morning Herald*, 7 March 1934, p. 23.
48 Butler, *Official History*, vol. III, p. 819.
49 Maxine Bucklow, 'Applied Psychology in Australia—the History' in M. Nixon and R. Taft (eds.), *Psychology in Australia: Achievements and Prospects*, Pergamon Press, Sydney, 1977, pp. 23–4.
50 Morris E. Miller, review, *Australian Journal of Psychology and Philosophy*, vol. IV, 1928, p. 232.
51 Garton, *The Cost of War*, p. 158.
52 Letter to the editor, *MJA*, 3 August 1935, p. 163. Butler's private files are full of leaflets and papers on eugenics and it was a regularly debated feature of Australia's national health of the day.
53 Butler, *Official History*, vol. III, table 57, p. 941.
54 Garton, *The Cost of War*, p. 167.
55 Butler, *Official History*, vol. III, p. 967.
56 Ibid., p. 823.
57 AWM 27 371/73 Part 1. In the smaller states, numbers were even lower. The West Australian Government estimated that there were approximately 25,000 ex-soldiers living in that state in 1928. 'The expectation of insanity among these is almost 1 to 1,700 per annum. This would mean that approximately 15 soldiers would be admitted per annum, of which about 30% would recover, which would leave a residue of about 10 per annum.' 'Medical Mental Hospitals ex-soldiers W.A.' D 394/1/4. NAA (Canberra). In 1936, of 139 males admitted to South Australia's Parkside Mental Hospital, only one patient's problems were attributable to 'war service' although another 86 men had causes 'unknown'. The same year, the Enfield Receiving House also recorded only one ex-military patient of 148 male patients. *Annual Report of the Inspector General of the Insane, South Australia, 1936*.

58 'Revision of Mental Patients', File SP948 G.530 NAA (Sydney).

59 Cyril Burt, *The Subnormal Mind*, Oxford University Press, 1937, p. 5.

60 There is little in the papers or published memoirs of senior AIF commanders, the likes of C. B. B. White, Monash, Elliot, and Gellibrand, that differs from Bean's assessment of the nation's soldiers. Their 'public' silence on the matter may have been a disservice to those who came to command the second AIF in 1939.

Chapter Nine
Observations and Reflections

The 'Great' War, the cataclysm of 1914–1918, stupefied its generation, but it also rattled men's psychological resilience in the face of unprecedented mental assault. It shook the military and the medical profession out of a complacent and condescending view of shell shock while reinvigorating, rather than inventing, the discipline of psychology which itself was boosted by the psychological challenges thrown up by the war. It had 'proved to be a historical moment at which the message started to seep through that there was something seriously awry with a science of psychiatry that had not put its moral relations in order by prizing equality and a willingness to show solidarity with its patients.'[1] Some scholars of postwar societies have suggested that the broader society will adapt in some instances to integrate and understand the wartime experience. But they, and 'specific elites therein can also erect barriers to protect their values, normal processes, vested interests and collective "sanity" from the potential moral anarchy of war—as reflected in war's actual victims, the veterans.'[2] This was certainly the case in Australia between 1918 and 1939. But it was a process marked more by variation and fluctuations in public opinion than it was by an abrupt and total rejection of the nation's war lunatics.

Despite the scars within Australian society, many of the lessons learned were forgotten by the eve of the Second World War, although the phrase 'shell shock' continued to retain its grip on the popular imagination. As late as 1943, one army psychiatrist was still advising against the use of the term. According to this doctor, 'medical officers were seeing at the base returned soldiers who allege that they were told by the regimental medical officer that they had "shell shock." We trust that this was untrue and that it was a fabrication of the patient's fertile imagination.'[3] Despite his admonitions, this officer, smug in his modernity, was content to quote the 1922 Shell Shock Commission and use its outmoded terminology.

In the broader Australian society there evolved two separate experiences when it came to remembering the war. The first included the official military panoply of commemoration and ceremonial that cemented the place of the 'digger' as a national icon. Judged on this alone, the life's work of Charles Bean had then been an outstanding success. The second was mostly hidden from public view or known only in family circles or local neighbourhoods. Away from the very public celebration of Australia's sacrifice to war were those soldiers who could not escape their own memories and experiences of the war—whether they had been shell shocked or not. Over time some were healed, while for others the passing years opened forgotten wounds. Ex-servicemen's clubs straddled both the military and the civilian worlds of their members. They were part of one while advocating for the other and there was always a tension between the two.

The shell shock crisis was something of a watershed in the psychiatric care of soldiers and, for the first time, removed a gender association from the term 'hysteria'. From 1914 to 1918 the military continued to view the problem as being the soldier's fault, aided by either his innate moral weakness or by a hereditary predisposition. Those other enemies of battle discipline, malingering and cowardice were, by association, added to an already heady mix of poorly understood neuroses. The establishment of a comprehensive repatriation system following the war assisted the mentally damaged soldier as it meant a concerted, if not always coordinated approach to his problems and a genuine concern to do the best by him as far as the army, his pension entitlements, and his medical treatment were concerned. But for many mentally scarred soldiers it would be a difficult return to civilian society. They returned as veterans and, as such, occupied an ambivalent position. There was then, as now, often a 'reciprocal suspicion and hostility...existing between the veteran and the civilian.'[4] They were not helped by some doctors' continuing to display a unique ambivalence to ex-service patients with psychological symptoms.

Postwar Australia also saw a number of developments, including mental and physical amenities and conditions of treatment, that had repercussions in civil practice, and extra-institutional organised endeavours to provide such. Unfortunately some of the same lessons had to be relearned after the Second World War, while others, such as the stigma of mental disease, would return earlier in 1940. Equally significantly but more concealed, was the war's contribution to the mental suffering and social cost to individuals and their families. Soldiers found their return to civilian life blighted by their front-line experiences, none of which could be appreciated or shared by their civilian counterparts—tragically, even by those closest to them. Between the wars there was, therefore, a public reluctance to discuss shell shock and a degree of impatience and frustration with soldiers' own struggle for 'normalcy'. This, together with increasingly stricter scrutiny of pensions by the Treasury, turned their dismay into anger.

By the late 1920s and 1930s, in Australia at least, there seems to have been a curious development when it came to identifying the incidence of 'true' shell shock among the war's mental wreckage. Figures from New South Wales (which are assumed to typify the broad demographics of the rest of the country) indicated that only 44 of the 327 ex-soldiers in that state's asylums who were inmates or out-patients were deemed by the authorities to have their insanity directly linked to war wounds, including 'shell concussion.'[5] There was also, from the victims' point of view, a regression in official thinking when it came to shell shock or war neuroses. A particularly interesting illustration of this concerns a surgeon who had expressed his concern that a patient who continued to suffer from shrapnel in situ in his body, was only now becoming 'depressed' about his condition and asked for a sympathetic hearing of his patient's case. The Deputy Commissioner of the Repatriation Commission took a different view and, in a throwback to 1915, issued the following statement: 'The examinations, arguments, improper revelation and discussion of medical matters and [the] search for evidence which arises from the present system of dealing with pension claims, fosters the development of the neurotic tendency as common in the community. Appalling examples come under my notice of the demoralisation of approximately normal useful individuals to a condition of *litigious invalidism*.'[6] The Deputy Commissioner simply grouped cases such as this man's among the mass of others claiming war pensions. In a word, he was totally unsympathetic.

Such an attitude seemed to hark back to what German psychologists had been saying during the First World War itself. The victim could not be trusted and his injuries were more suited to being viewed as industrial rather than military in nature. Whether the Commissioner's views reflected frustration at the continued poor press suffered by his department or the ongoing advocacy of the ex-servicemen's groups is unclear.

War neuroses had a significant impact on families and the hitherto traditional family roles and values. The 1920s also saw suppressed or forgotten war memories emerge among ex-servicemen, a trend which worsened with the deteriorating economic climate. Generally the repatriation system was immune to the lack of funds that plagued the state's asylum system and continued to assist ex-soldier mental casualties.[7] Ex-servicemen's associations and individual politicians also continued to lobby for support and recognition of their colleagues. But many returned soldiers had been won over to Bean's view of the war and their own place in it. In espousing this view they unwittingly pushed the war neurotic into the background before the wider public and political delicacy consigned them to oblivion.

While making no claim to clinical expertise, it is difficult in a work such as this to ignore the subsequent psychological history of the Australian military. Mental problems under the guise of a spectrum of diagnostic names have been scrutinised and discussed publicly in a way never before seen in Australia. The problems of Australia's Vietnam veterans and, more recently, those deployed to the various Gulf and Middle East conflicts of recent times, provide evidence of this. Questions are invariably asked of links between shell shock and, for example, PTSD. Some scholars have questioned whether shell shock was really PTSD. While some believe that it is, others caution against identifying PTSD with the experiences of 1914–1918, arguing that this disorder 'is not so much a truth that has been discovered, as an invention or strategic fiction.'[8] Parallels such as these also risk ignoring the fundamental suffering of these soldiers—both physically and psychologically. It is worth remembering that the traumatic memory is a human construction: 'It originates in the scientific and clinical discourses of the nineteenth century, before that time, there is unhappiness, despair and disturbing recollections, but no traumatic meaning in the sense that we know it today.'[9]

On the one hand Harold Merskey has suggested that 'post-traumatic stress disorder represents very well the response which was once called "shell shock" in soldiers, as well as an effect of other conditions in causing stress (e.g. frightening accidents). However there is no less evidence of gross conversion symptoms than was found with shell shock.'[10] A senior Australian medical officer also believes that this disorder 'is caused by a psychologically traumatic event that is generally outside the range of normal human experience, resulting in symptoms of acute mental and physical distress.'[11] The symptoms he lists include intensive flashbacks; emotional dissociation; psychological numbing; arousal of fear; depression; and substance abuse. The experiences of the Australian soldier in the First World War neatly fall into both views on the subject. In this respect the diggers of old share something tragically unique with some of their modern-day counterparts. The difference is that, in the twenty-first century, there is a recognition not only that psychological injury actually exists, but that soldiers are no less men for their psychological experiences.

However this sharing has yet to spill over to the long-held collective and official memory of the Great War—the sanitised, sane and heroic image of nation created by Bean. There is, of course, an inconsistency here. Why did the majority of ex-servicemen acquiesce in a public recollection of war that had so many omissions? Alistair Thompson has proposed that, although Bean's 'articulation of Anzac identity was more homogenous and nationalistic than the varieties of Anzac experience, the Anzacs did not reject his definition of Australian military manhood because they shared a substantial common understanding of what it meant to be an Australian soldier.'[12] Perhaps this fitted well with their self-image and at the same time masked self-doubt and repressed memories. Other scholars have argued that Australia's response to its ex-soldiers was overwhelmingly parsimonious and self-serving.[13] But this was not the case in their treatment of most soldiers, although the marginalised war neurotics were early victims of the deteriorating economy and a social re-assessment of both their contribution to the war and the authenticity of their metal suffering.

Some writers have suggested that Britain never recovered from the shock of the 1914–18 war. The 'war poets and novelists who wrote of "shell-shock" provided a poetic way of making that point.'[14] In Australia it was the likes of C.E.W. Bean and protègès such as A.G. Butler who did the same through denying shell shock its place in the collective memory both of Australians who were psychologically affected by that war and those who witnessed it from afar—either in time or space. At the same time the increasing popularity of commemorations such as Anzac Day signals the replacement of traditional symbols such as the Church and loyalty to the Crown as the public struggles to find and then identify with suitable national rituals and images. Historian E. M. Andrews' call in 1993 to look at the Anzac myth 'with clear [and one might add, dry] eyes' remains largely unheeded.[15]

Despite Bean's editing, his official war history still allowed ex-servicemen and women positive ways to make sense of their wartime experience. However, by producing an account that generalised the Anzac experience according 'to the themes of national identity and achievement, and that marginalised war experiences that did not fit those themes, Bean's official history played an influential role in shaping the ways in which ex-servicemen articulated their own war experiences and identified themselves as Anzacs.'[16] The same may be said of Butler's medical history of the First World War. Both men had seen life at the front for themselves but had interpreted what they saw in a way that would not bring their fellow soldiers into 'disrepute'. Bean and Butler shared similar middle class values and backgrounds and both had a vision for the new nation. The popularity of their works, particularly Bean with his fine turn of phrase, helps to explain why there was so little visibility of the war neurotic in Australia during the interwar years. While 'shell shock' as a term, even a metaphor, for the tragedy of the Great War is still evocative, any real understanding of its impact on individuals has perhaps been thwarted.

Since 1918 later generations have been better 'immunised' to the horrors of war than their forebears, few of whom had much exposure to horror or even to the products and systems of heavy industry. The centrality of the 'industrial' aspect of the First World War is a common theme in many works on shell shock. Peter Leese has suggested that one reason for the potency of the memory of shell shock is that it became 'the first and most powerful expression of the destructive effects of industrial warfare on the mind, of the war generation's tragedy.'[17] From the military perspective, later large-scale conflicts were generally more mobile and manoeuverist than the stalemate along the Western Front and hence there was less 'classic' shell shock seen than was evident in the period 1915–1918. Others have asked the question 'was this industrialized war and its scale of technologically administered violence beyond mere human endurance? If the answer was "yes", then neurosis was an inevitable, even normal consequence of the enormous, invisible threats focused upon those huddled in the trench system.'[18] Shell shock and neuroses then become part of the fabric not only of the real war, but also of the war remembered. Yet these neurotic soldiers remain outside of, and apart from, the myth as it has evolved. Madness and the military are still seen as poles apart, but in reality there is a perverse relationship between the two—the one is a cause, the other a consequence.

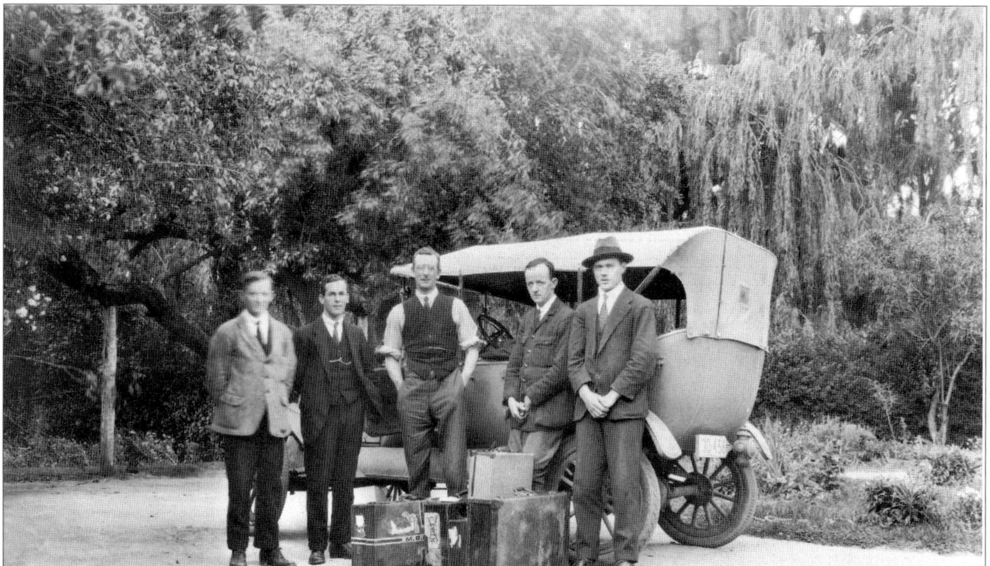

Journalist cum historian Charles Bean (third from the left) and colleagues with material for the first volume of his seminal history of the First World War. Canberra, 12 December 1920.
His was very much an optimistic view of nation-building.
(AWM A05383)

It seems that subsequent generations of 'war mad' would be also doomed to marginalisation. During the Second World War the myths of the first 'diggers' were 'authenticated and perpetuated' demonstrating that 'Anzac was no pejorative "myth" at all.'[19] Soldiers who have been scarred mentally by the profession of arms seem still to struggle for a place in Australia's perception of the nation's military tradition. Bean's artificial construct of the Anzac myth continues within our society today, as does the exclusion of the shell-shocked soldier. Despite his role as a life-long supporter of Australian soldiers there is little evidence that Charles Bean attempted to revisit the issue of war neurotics at any time from 1918 until his death in 1968. Perhaps his true feelings towards the shell-shocked soldier are revealed by his rejection of the following poem, one of many sent to Bean for publication in his *Anzac Book*. Was Trooper McCarthy's a forlorn hope?

'...When Lone Pine [Gallipoli] is a memory, that's slipping from us fast,
And Killd Bahr's becoming a nightmare from the past,
When we have left the trenches, and the dugouts on the hill.
Each heart will leap as never, we thought men's hearts could thrill.
Away from horrid memories of death moans and of pain...'[20]

Trooper E. P. McCarthy, 6th Light Horse

Endnotes

1 Barham, 'Forgotten Lunatics of the Great War', p. 365.
2 Dean, 'War and Psychiatry', p. 65.
3 Bostock and Jones, *The Nervous Soldier*, p. 43.
4 Dean, 'War and Psychiatry', p. 81.
5 'Revision of Mental Cases', 4 July 1938, SP948 G530 NAA (Sydney).
6 'Neurasthenia' Memorandum from the Deputy Commissioner to the Secretary of the Repatriation Commission, 11 March 1937. SP948/1 G1022. NAA (Sydney).
7 Despite the popular view of the Commission as being antipathetic to these men, it held to its mandate right through to the next war. In May 1946 it established a high-powered special medical advisory committee to ensure the best possible medical care for those suffering 'physically or mentally as a result of their war service.' 'Special Advisory Committee, Medical Services of the Repatriation Department'. File: 39 NAA (Sydney).
8 Barham, 'Forgotten Lunatics of the Great War', p. 367, quoting Allan Young, *Harmony of Illusions*.
9 Allan Young, *The Harmony of Illusions: Inventing Post-Traumatic Stress Disorder*, Princeton, 1995, p. 141.
10 Merskey, 'Shell-Shock', pp. 263–4.
11 Warfe, 'Post Traumatic stress and the Australian Defence Force', p. 86.

12 Thompson, *Anzac Memories*, p. 70.

13 However this author agrees with Lloyd Robson's assessment of the government at that time: 'it is difficult to imagine any nation offering its ex-soldiers more or holding them and their values in higher esteem.' Robson, 'The Australian Soldier: Formation of a Stereotype', p. 330.

14 Winter, 'Shell-shock and the Cultural History of the Great War', p.10.

15 Andrews, *The Anzac Illusion*, p. 215.

16 Thompson, *Anzac Memories*, p. 156.

17 Leese, *Shell Shock*, p. 176.

18 Leed, *No Man's Land*, p. 180.

19 Robin Gerster, *Big Noting: The Heroic Theme in Australian War Writing*, Melbourne University Press, 1987, p. 172.

20 Segment of a poem submitted by Trooper E. P. McCarthy, 6th Australian Light Horse, 2 December 1915, AWM 1362. This poem was one of many rejected by C.E.W. Bean during the compilation of his *Anzac Book*.

Appendix

Appendix

Two interesting pieces of correspondence testify to the caution with which psychological statistics for World War I need to be treated. One of the military players in this psychological drama, J. W. Springthorpe, confided to Butler after the war that, with respect to 'statistics [shell shock, 'flu, etc.] I can hardly see how they can do anything but seriously mislead.' Diagnoses were almost routinely made at hospitals by a junior admitting officer, partly on the scanty notes from RMOs who themselves 'had neither time nor competence to disentangle symptoms from disease or to attribute true causation or to state the actual, even dominating facts.' Pointedly, he added that it 'was more what was omitted than what was noted that really mattered in numerable cases.'[1]

In correspondence dated 16 May 1940, Butler described the loss of all Australian clinical records (which were coded and remarkably comprehensive) which were burned in London shortly after the Armistice. He discussed the unreliability of the Australian (and UK) statistics and also stated: 'For the rest we have, as individual groups, those of "hysterical" types; those of "neurasthenia" and "psychasthenic" types and "secondary neuroses". The latter includes all the states developing as [a] result of secondary "motives"—as one may say; as the desire to escape war service during the war, and to obtain a pension during the peace—with the infinite variation in motivation from deliberate and conscious engineering to the most primitive organic or instinctive compulsion...'[2]

Casualty Admissions to the 7th Australian Field Ambulance.[3]

This table is included to provide an idea of the fluidity of psychological casualty figures depending on hostile activity at the front. The success of a 'common sense' approach to managing such casualties, even by 1916, can also be seen in the numbers ultimately evacuated from their units to casualty clearing stations at the rear.

Date	Number	% shell shock to all Admissions	% Discharged to CCS
28 July 1916	11	30	100
29 July	29	45	38
30 July	38	77	42
1 Aug 1916	24	90	30
2	5	71	40
3	12	80	45
4	4	33	0
5	5	28	20
6	33	45	30
7	47	49	15
8	137	71	48
9	107	66	26
10	69	55	17
11	74	75	15
12	130	98	7

Comparative data on Pensions Expenditure (including dependants) 1930s:[4]

	Per 1,000 population £	Per 1,000 enlistments £	Population (m)
British Empire	11,538	98.684	65
France	11,494	58,743	41.5
Germany	10,303	52,037	66
U.S.A	4,844	122,960	122
Australia	11,051	180,691	6.8

Classification of Disabilities of Australian War Pensioners[5]

	'War Neurosis'	Total Pensioners	%
1924	2,603	72,760	3.57
1925	2,543	72,128	3.52
1926	2,554	72,128	3.54
1927	2,583	72,388	3.56
1928	2,624	72,667	3.61
1929	2,727	73,436	3.71
1930	2,820	74,587	3.78
1931	2,908	75,316	3.86
1932	2,949	75,646	3.89
1933	2,951	75,244	3.92
1934	2,959	75,037	3.94
1935	3,014	74,998	4.01
1936	3,147	76,337	4.12
1937	3,240	77,076	4.20
1938	3,328	77,315	4.30
1939	3,345	77,151	4.33
1940	3,311	76,462	4.33

The number of 'mental cases under restraint'—i.e. independently of those treated at home, and those not accepted as of war causation, rose from 341 in 1924 to 513 in 1940, an increase of just over fifty per cent. Letter from C. K. Parkinson MC (formerly a Lieutenant-Colonel in the AAMC and Senior Medical Boarding Officer) to A. G. Butler, 5 November 1935. At that time he was the Senior Medical Officer (NSW) for the Repatriation Department.[6]

Mortality rate of war pensioners with major psychoses (1922–1931)[7]:

Year	No. of Pensioners	Deaths	Year	No. of Pensioners	Deaths
1922	444	9	1927	627	14
1923	449	12	1928	674	21
1924	468	14	1929	691	9
1925	492	10	1930	789	12
1926	584	14	1931	859	9

Endnotes

1 Letter from J.W. Springthorpe to A.G. Butler, 20 July 1923. AWM 41 [2008].
2 Letter from A.G. Butler to Major S.O. Cowen (Department of Defence) AWM 41 [282].
3 Source: SECRET Letter to DMS 4th Army from Lieutenant-Colonel H. B. Sawer for Surgeon General Slogett, HQ 4th Army, 17 November 1916. AWM 41 649.
4 Butler, *Official History*, vol. III, p. 962.
5 Ibid., p. 965.
6 AWM 41 [54].
7 Ibid., p. 834.

Bibliography

Primary Sources

National Archives of Australia
Canberra:
A 458 E.368/9, A 2489/1/1920/1739, A 2487/1/1921/9338, A 2487/1922/13913, A 2487 B18/7061, A 2489.20/1447, A458.Q 356/19, A 2487.1922/9833, A 248.20/1447, A 458 745/1/339, A 2487.1921/9338, A 458.0368/5, A 2483 B.18/4076, A 3280.P7945, A 457.AK403/6, A11804.1922/605, A 458.K368/5, D 394/1/4/, G394/1/4.

Sydney:
SP 9481/1 G900, SP 9481/1 G530, G900 Part 1, SP 9481/1 G530, SP 9481/1 G1022, SP 459/1/471/1/299, G39; and G188.

State Records of New South Wales:
Broughton Hall Psychiatric Clinic Files 14/8956–78, 14/8979–80, 14/8981–9098, Case Papers (Australian Military Forces) 1915–1920, 14/8956–78.

Australian War Memorial, Canberra:
AWM 11 1507/24/2, AWM 16 4364/29/1, AWM 25 85/8, AWM 25 885/1–5, AWM 25 885/7, AWM 25 399/28, AWM 27 304/29, AWM 27 310/78, AWM 27 371/73 Part 1, AWM 27 376/215, AWM 27 76/216, AWM 27 376/213, AWM 32 /61, AWM 32 /62, AWM 32 /63, AWM 41 /291, AWM 41 /483, AWM 41 /279, AWM 41 /285, AWM 41 /290, AWM 41 /474, AWM 41 /657, AWM 41 /658, AWM 41 /659, AWM 41 /934, AWM 41 /740, AWM 41 /290, AWM 41 /737, AWM 41 26/48, AWM 41/2015, AWM 44 16/4 Parts 1, 2, 3; AWM 253 AIF 498/1/693, AWM 243 AIF498/1/693.

Mitchell Library of New South Wales, Sydney:
Barwick, A. A. ML MSS 1493
Brookes, J. ML MSS 2908
Colley-Priest, L. ML MSS 2439
De Mouncy, E. ML MSS 1839
Faulkner, G.R. ML MSS 1151
Moore, A.J. ML MSS 911
Sillas, E.L. ML MSSS 1840
Watson, W.C. ML MSS 2949

Secondary Sources

Unpublished Thesis
Richard Lindstrom, 'The Australian Experience of Psychological Casualties in War 1915-1939'. Thesis submitted for the Degree of Doctor of Philosophy, Department of Humanities, Faculty of Arts, Victoria University of Technology, February 1997.

Newspapers and Magazines
Argus
Aussie
Australian Worker
Bulletin
New York Times
Repatriation
Reveille
Rising Sun
Sydney Morning Herald
Smith's Weekly
Sydney Sun
The Times

Journal Articles
Anon., 'Naval and Military News', *Medical Journal of Australia*, 16 January 1915, p.58.
Adrian, E.D. and Yealland, L.R., 'Treatment of Some Common War Neuroses', *Lancet*, 9 June 1917, pp. 867–72.
Bean, C.E.W., 'Our War History', *Bulletin*, 27 May 1942, p. 2.
Beattie-Smith, W., 'Address in Neurology and Psychiatry', Ninth Session, Australasian Medical Congress, Sydney, 1911, *Australasian Medical Gazette*, 20 October 1911, pp. 561–65.
Beattie-Smith, W. and Powys, A.O., 'Insanity in Victoria and New South Wales', *Australasian Medical Gazette*, 20 June 1906, pp.288–9.
Bogacz, T., 'War Neurosis and Cultural Change in England 1914-1922: the Work of the War Office Committee of Enquiry into "Shell-Shock"', *Journal of Contemporary History*, 24, 1989, pp. 27–56.
Book reviews, 'Shell Concussion and Shell Shock' and 'War Neuroses', *Medical Journal of Australia*, 1 March 1919, p.173.
Bourke, J., 'Shell Shock and the Australian Soldiers in the Great War', *Sabretache*, vol. XXXVI, no. 3, July-September 1995, pp. 3–10.
Bucklow, M., 'Applied Psychology in Australia – the History', in Nixon, M., and Taft, R. (eds.), *Psychology in Australia: Achievements and Prospects*, Pergamon Press, Sydney, 1977, pp. 23–9.
Butler, A.G., 'The Treatment of "The Effort Syndrome"', *Medical Journal of Australia*, 31 May 1941, pp. 667–8.
Campbell, A.W., 'Remarks on some Neuroses and Psychoses in War', *Medical Journal of Australia*, 15 April 1916, pp. 319–23.
Cooter, R., 'War and Modern Medicine' in Bynum, W. F., and Porter, R. (eds.), *Encyclopaedia of Modern Medicine*, London, 1993.
——, 'Malingering in Modernity: Psychological Scripts and Adversarial Encounters during the First World War' in Cooter, R., Harrison, M., and Sturdy, S. (eds.), *War, Medicine and Modernity*, Stroud, 1999.
Cooter, R., and Sturdy, S., 'Of War, Medicine and Modernity: An Introduction' in: Cooter, R., Harrison, M., and Sturdy, S. (eds.), *War Medicine and Modernity*, Stroud, 1999.
Coupland Winn, R., 'Psychology in Relation to Modern Medical Practice', *Medical Journal of Australia*, 6 December 1930, pp. 753–8.

——, Psychoanalysis and General Practice', *Medical Journal of Australia*, 29 February 1936, pp. 293–9.

Dane, P., 'The Psycho-Neuroses of Soldiers and Their Treatment', *Medical Journal of Australia*, 25 April 1925, pp. 427–30.

——, 'Traumatic Psychoneurosis', *Medical Journal of Australia*, 25 February1950, pp. 266–7.

——, 'Psychoanalysis and Psychotherapy' in *MJA*, December 1926.

Dean, E. T., 'War and Psychiatry: examining the diffusion theory in light of the insanity defence in post-World War I Britain', in *History of Psychiatry*, vol. IV, 1993, pp. 61–82.

Downey, M. H., 'The Management and Treatment of Early Insanity', a paper read before the South Australian Branch of the British Medical Association and published in the *Australasian Medical Gazette*, 20 December 1911, pp. 719–24.

Editorial: 'Lunacy Reform in Victoria', *Australasian Medical Gazette*, 20 June 1906, pp. 288–9.

Editorial: 'Research in Psychiatry', *Medical Journal of Australia*, 17 March 1917, pp.231–2.

Editorial: 'The Wastage from Incompleteness', *Medical Journal of Australia*, 22 July 1916, pp. 59–60.

Editorial: 'The Mental Hospitals of New South Wales', *Medical Journal of Australia*, 27 April 1935, pp. 529–30.

Editorial: 'The Psychological Approach', *Medical Journal of Australia*, 20 August 1938, pp. 289–90.

Godfrey, C.G., 'Some Cases of Stammering from War Shock treated by Psychotherapy', *Medical Journal of Australia*, 28 September 1918, pp.262–4.

Fennell, S., 'Psychiatry in New Zealand 1912-1948' in Brookes, B., and Thomson, J. (eds.), *Unfortunate Folk: Essays on Mental Health Trends in New Zealand 1863-1992*, University of Otago, 2001, pp. 136–152.

Feudtner, C., 'Minds the Dead Have Ravished: Shell Shock, History and the Evolution of Disease Systems', *History of Science*, 31, Part 4, no. 94, 1993, pp. 377–420.

Finlay-Jones, R., 'The Effect of War on Theory and Practice of Psychiatry in Australia', Attwood, H. et al. (eds.), *Patients, Practitioners and Techniques*, 2nd National Conference in Medicine and Health in Australia, University of Melbourne, 1985, pp. 43–53.

Fraser, A.C., 'Notes on three Cases of Functional Disease of the Nervous System seen during the Voyage from England to Australia', *Medical Journal of Australia*, 22 November 1919, pp. 436–7.

Griffith, P., 'Fighting Spirit: Leadership, Morale on the "empty battlefield" of the future' in Evans, M., and Ryan, A. (eds.), *The Human Face of War: Killing, Fear and Chaos in Battle*, Allen & Unwin, Sydney, 2000.

Grossman, D., 'Human Factors in War: the psychology and physiology of close combat' in John Keegan, *The Face of War*, Jonathan Cape, London, 1977.

Haywood, R., Review of P. Leese, *Shell Shock* (2002), in *Journal of Contemporary History*, vol. 40, 2005, p.169.

Jones, E. and Wessely, S., 'Psychiatric Battle Casualties: an Intra- and Interwar Comparison', *British Journal of Psychiatry*, vol. 178, 2001, pp. 242–7.

Jones, S. E., 'Experiences in the Treatment of Voluntary Patients at the Psychiatric Clinic, Broughton Hall', *Medical Journal of Australia*, 4 September 1926, pp. 316–19.

Jones, W.E., 'Case of Shell Shock', *Medical Journal of Australia*, 4 March 1916, pp. 203–4.

Kent, D., 'The Anzac Book and the Anzac legend: C.E.W. Bean as Editor and Image Maker', *Historical Studies*, vol. 21, no. 84, April 1985, pp. 376–390.

Kosky, R., 'From Morality to Madness: A Reappraisal of the Asylum Movement in Psychiatry 1800-1940', *Australian and New Zealand Journal of Psychiatry*, vol. 20, 1986, pp.180–7.

Leese, P., 'Why are they not cured? British Shellshock Treatment During the Great War' in Micale, M. S., and Lerner, P. (eds.), *Traumatic Pasts: History, Psychiatry and Trauma in the Modern Age, 1870-1930*, Cambridge, 2001.

Lengwiler, M., 'Psychiatry beyond the Asylum: the origins of German Military Psychiatry before Word War I' in *History of Psychiatry*, vol. 14, 2001, pp. 41–62.

Lerner, P., 'Psychiatry and Casualties of War in Germany, 1914-18', *Journal of Contemporary History*, 35 (1), 2000, pp.13–28.

Lowson, J.P., 'Some Points in the Psychology of Nervous Breakdown', *Australian Journal of Psychology and Philosophy*, vol. II, 1924, pp.113–35.

——, 'The Treatment of War Neuroses by Abreaction of the War Shock', *Medical Journal of Australia*, 6 November 1926, pp. 621–6.

McWhae, D.M., 'Neuroses', *Medical Journal of Australia*, 2 October 1920, pp. 337–42.

Merskey, H., 'Shell-Shock' in Freeman, H., and Berrios, G.E. (eds.), *150 Years of British Psychiatry*, vol. I, London, 1991.

Miller, E. M., review of F.C. Bartlett's 'Psychology and the Soldier', *Australian Journal of Psychology and Philosophy*, vol. IV, 1928, pp. 231–2.

Minogue, S.J., 'Suicides Amongst returned Soldiers of the 1914-1918 War', *Medical Journal of Australia*, 24 February 1945, pp. 195–8.

Morgan, I., 'Hypnotic Suggestion' *Medical Journal of Australia*, 15 January 1927, pp. 85–92.

Mosse, G., 'Shell-shock as social disease', *Journal of Contemporary History*, 35 (1), 2000, pp. 101–8.

Myers, C., '"Contributions to the Study of Shell Shock" being an Account of Certain Cases treated by Hypnosis', *Lancet*, vol. II, 8 January 1916, pp. 65–9.

Ørner, R. J., 'Post-Traumatic Stress Disorders and European War Veterans', *British Journal of Clinical Psychiatry*,' vol. 31, 1992, pp.387–403.

Pern, S., 'A Plea for Adequate Recognition of the Part that can be played in Shell–shock by Septic Foci', *Medical Journal of Australia*, 10 August 1918, pp.15–16.

Pierce, B., 'Shell shock', *The Medical Annual*, Wright, Bristol, 1917, pp. 461–6.

Ramsay-Hunt, J., 'Neurasthenia in Soldiers', *The Medical Annual*, Wright, Bristol, 1916, pp. 479–84.

Regnell, W.R., 'The Psychoneuroses of War', *Medical Journal of Australia*, 7 June 1919, pp. 455–460.

Reid, F., 'Playing the Game to the Army: The Royal Army Medical Corps, Shell Shock and the Great War', in *War & Society*, vol. 23, no.1, May 2005, pp. 61–86.

Report, *Medical Journal of Australia*, 25 September 1920, pp. 324–5.

Report, *Medical Journal of Australia*, 7 June 1919, pp. 472–3.

Report, 'The Treatment of "Neurasthenia" in Soldiers', *Medical Journal of Australia*, 7 December 1918, pp. 480–1.

Robson, L., 'The Australian Soldier: Formation of a Stereotype' in McKernan, M., and Browne, M. (eds.), *Australia: Two Centuries of War and Peace*, Australian War Memorial and Allen & Unwin, Canberra, 1988.

Samuels, A., 'Invisible Wounds' in *Repatriation*, 25 June 1919.

Shepherd, B., 'The Early Treatment of Mental Disorders': R.G. Rowes and Maghull 1914-1918' in Freeman, H., and Berrios, G.E.(eds.), *150 Years of British Psychiatry*, vol. II: *The Aftermath*, London, 1996.

——, 'Shell-shock' in Freeman, H. (ed.), *A Century of Psychiatry*, London, 1999.
Springthorpe, J.W., 'Twelve Months' Service at the Front', *Medical Journal of Australia*, 29 April 1916, pp. 1–8.
——, 'War Neuroses and Civil Practice', *Medical Journal of Australia*, 4 October 1919, pp. 279–84.
Stone, M., 'Shellshock and the Psychiatrists' in Bynum, W.F., Porter, R., and Shepherd, M. (eds.), *The Anatomy of Madness*, vol. II, London, 1985.
Summons, W., 'Medical Work seen in the Australian Military Hospitals', *Medical Journal of Australia*, 22 September 1917, pp. 244–7.
The Rising Sun, no. 2, vol. II, Sydney, December 1928.
Thomson, M., 'Status, Manpower and Mental Fitness: Mental Deficiency in the First World War', in Cooter, R., Harrison, M., and Sturdy, S. (eds.), *War, Medicine and Modernity* (Stroud, 1999).
Turner, W.A., 'Arrangements for the Care of Cases of Nervous and Mental Shock Coming from Overseas', *The Lancet*, 27 May 1916, pp.1073–5.
Warfe, P., 'Post Traumatic stress and the Australian Defence Force: Lessons from peace operations in Rwanda and Lebanon', in Evans, M., and Ryan, A. (eds.), *The Human Face of War: Killing, Fear and Chaos in Battle*, Allen & Unwin, Sydney, 2000.
Weaver, J., and Wright, D., 'Shell Shock and the Politics of Asylum Committal in New Zealand, 1916-22', *Health and History*, vol.7, no.1, 2005, pp.17–40.
Wessely, S., Review of Paul Lerner's 'Hysterical Men: War, Psychiatry and the Politics of Germany 1890-1930', *History of Psychiatry*, vol.15, issue 4, no.60, December 2004, pp. 490–5.
White, B., Combat Stress Reaction, *Defence Force Journal*, no.55, 1985, p. 26.
Wiltshire, H., 'A Contribution to the Etiology of Shell Shock', *The Lancet*, vol. II, 17 June 1916, pp. 1207–12.
Winter, J.M., 'Shell-shock and the Cultural History of the Great War', *Journal of Contemporary History*, 35, 2000, pp. 7–11.

Books:
Ahrenfeldt, R., *Psychiatry in the British Army in the Second World War*, Routledge & Keegan Paul, London, 1958.
Allen, J. A., *Sex and Secrets: Crimes Involving Australian Women since 1880*, Oxford University Press, Melbourne, 1990.
Andrews, E.M., *The Anzac Illusion: Anglo-Australian Relations during World War 1*, Cambridge University Press, Melbourne, 1993.
Barham, P., *Forgotten Lunatics of the Great War*, Yale Press, London, 2004.
Barrett, J. W., *A Vision of the Possible*, H.K. Lewis, London, 1919.
——, *The Australian Army Medical Corps in Egypt*, H.K. Lewis, London, 1918.
Bartov, *Omer Murder in Our Midst: The Holocaust, Industrial Killing and Representation*, Oxford University Press, New York, 1996.
Bassett, J., *Guns and Brooches*, Oxford University Press, Melbourne, 1992.
Bean, C.E.W., *The Story of Anzac*, University of Queensland Press, reprint 1981.
Binneveld, H., *From Shell Shock to Combat Stress: A Comparative History of Military Psychiatry*, Amsterdam University Press, 1997.
Blaikie, G., *Remember Smith's Weekly?*, Rigby, Sydney, 1966.
Blair, D., *Dinkum Diggers: an Australian Battalion*, Melbourne University Press, 2001.
Bostock, J. and E. Jones, *The Nervous Soldier: A Handbook for the Prevention, Detection and Treatment of Nervous Inability in War*, Queensland University Press, Brisbane, 1943.

Bourke, J., *Dismembering the Male: Men's Bodies, Britain and the Great War*, Reakton, London, 1996.

——, *An Intimate History of Killing: Face-to-Face Combat in Twentieth Century Warfare*, Grantor Books, London, 1999.

Burt, C., *The Subnormal Mind*, Oxford University Press, 1937.

Butler, A. G., *Gallipoli, Palestine and New Guinea, The Official History of the Australian Army Medical Services in the War of 1914-18*, vol.1, Australian War Memorial, Canberra, 1930.

——, *The Western Front, The Official History of the Australian Army Medical Services in the War of 1914-18*, vol. II, Australian War Memorial, Canberra, 1940.

——, *Problems and Services, The Australian Army Medical Services in the War of 1914-18*, vol. III, Australian War Memorial, Canberra, 1943.

——, *The Digger: A Study in Democracy*, Angus & Robertson, Sydney, 1945.

Bynum, W., *Anatomy of Madness*, Tavistock, London, 1988.

Carberry, A. D., *The New Zealand Medical Service in the Great War 1914-1918*, Whitecombe & Tombs, Wellington, 1924.

Carney, T. and Hanks, P., *Social Security in Australia*, Oxford University Press, Melbourne, 1994.

Cohen, D., *The War Came Home: Disabled Veterans in Britain and Germany, 1914-1939*, Berkeley, 2001.

Coleburne, C. and Makinnon, D. (eds.), *Madness in Australia: histories, heritage and asylum*, Queensland University Press, 2003.

Cooter, R., *Surgery and Society in Peace and War: Orthopaedics and the Organisation of Modern Medicine, 1880–1948*, London, 1993.

Corns, C., and Hughes-Wilson, J., *Blindfold and Alone: British Military Executions in the Great War*, London, 2001.

Damousi, J., *Freud in the Antipodes: A Cultural History of Psychology in Australia*, University of NSW Press, Sydney, 2005.

——, *Living with the Aftermath*, Cambridge University Press, Melbourne, 2001.

——, *The Labour of Loss: Mourning, Memory and Wartime*, Cambridge University Press, Melbourne, 1999.

Deane, E., *Shook Over Hell*, Harvard University Press, Mass., 1997.

Eder, M.D., *War Shock*, W. Heinemann, London, 1917.

Edwards, A.T., *Patients are People*, Currajong, Sydney, 1968.

Ellery, R.S., *The Cow Jumped over the Moon: Private papers of a Psychiatrist*, F.W. Cheshire, Melbourne, 1956.

Evans, M., and Ryan, A. (eds.), *The Human Face of War: Killing, Fear and Chaos in Battle*, Allen & Unwin, Sydney, 2000.

Fromkin, D., *Europe's Last Summer: Why the World went to War in 1914*, Heinemann, London, 2004.

Gammage, B., *The Broken Years: Australian Soldiers in the Great War*, Australian National University, Canberra, 1975.

Garton, S., *Medicine and Madness: A Social History of Insanity in New South Wales 1880-1940*, University of New South Wales Press, Sydney, 1988.

——, *The Cost of War: Australians Return*, Oxford, 1996.

Gerster, R., *Big Noting: The Heroic Theme in Australian War Writing*, Melbourne University Press, 1987.

Gijswijt-Hofstra, M., and Porter, R. (eds.), *Cultures of Neurasthenia from Beard to the First World War*, Amsterdam, 2001.

Heseltine, H. (ed.), *The Shock of Battle*, Occasional Paper, no.16, ADFA, Canberra, 1989.
Holden, W., *Shell Shock*, Channel 4 Books, London, 1998.
Jones, K., *Asylums and After: a Revised History of the Mental Health Services from the Early 18th Century to the Late 1990s*, Athlone, London, 1939.
James, W., *The Australian Army Medical Corps in Egypt*, H.K. Lewis, London, 1918.
Laffin, J., *Damn the Dardanelles*, Sun Papermac, Melbourne, 1985.
Lake, M., *The Limits of Hope: Soldier Settlement in Victoria 1915-1938*, Oxford University Press, Melbourne, 1987.
Leed, E., *NoMan's Land: Combat and Identity in World War One*, Cambridge, 1979.
Leese, P., *Shell Shock: Traumatic Neurosis and the British Soldiers of the First World War*, London, 2002.
Lewis, T., *The Soldier's heart and the Effort Syndrome*, 2nd edition, Shaw & Sons, London, 1940.
Lewis, M., *Managing Madness: psychiatry and society in Australia 1788-1980*, AGPS Press, Canberra, 1988.
Lloyd, C., and J. Rees, *The Last Shilling: A History of Repatriation in Australia*, Melbourne University Press, 1994.
MacCurdy, J. T., *War Neuroses*, Cambridge, 1918.
McMullin, R., *Pompey Elliot*, Scribe, Melbourne, 2002.
MacPhail, A., *Official History of the Canadian Forces in the Great War 1914-1919: the Medical Services*, Acland, Ottawa, 1925.
MacPherson, W.G. (ed.), *History of the Great War Based On Official Documents: Medical Services, General History*, vol.1, H.M.S.O., London, 1921.
MacPherson, W.G., Herringham, W.P., Elliott, T.R., and Balfour, A. (eds.), *History of the Great War Based on Official Documents: Diseases of the War*, vol. II, London, 1923.
Mitchell, T.J. and Smith, G., *History of the Great War based On Official Documents. Medical Services: Casualties and Medical Statistics of the Great War*, London, 1931.
Moore, W., *The Thin Yellow Line*, Cooper Ltd., London, 1974.
Mott, F.W., *War Neuroses and Shell-Shock*, London, 1919.
Nixon, M., and Taft, R. (eds.), *Psychology in Australia: Achievements and Prospects*, Pergamon Press, Sydney, 1977.
O'Keefe, B., *Medicine at War: Medical Aspects of Australia's Involvement in Southeast Asian Conflicts 1950-1972*, Allen & Unwin, Sydney, 1994.
Oppenheim, J., *Shattered Nerves: Doctors, Patients and Depression in Victorian England*, Oxford, 1991.
Pugsley, C., *The Face of Hell: New Zealanders and Military Discipline in the First World War*, Hodder & Stoughton, Auckland, 1991.
Prior, R. and Wilson, T., *The Somme*, University of New South Wales Press, Sydney, 2005.
Raftery, J., *Marks of War*, Lythrum Press, Adelaide, 2003.
Ramsay, R.J. (ed.), *Hell, Hope and Heroes: Life in the Field Ambulance in World War 1*, Rosenberg, Dural, 2005.
Read, C. S., *Military Psychiatry in Peace and War*, London, 1920.
Ross, J., *The Myth of the Digger: The Australian Soldier in Two World Wars*, Hale & Iremonger, Sydney, 1985.
Ross, T.A., Lectures on War Neuroses, Edward Arnold, London, 1941.
Seal, G., *Inventing Anzac: The Digger and National Mythology*, University of Queensland, 2004.
Shepherd, B., *A War of Nerves: Soldiers and Psychiatrists, 1914-1994*, London, 2000.

Showalter, E., *The Female Malady: Women, Madness and English Culture 1830 –1980*, Pantheon, New York, 1985.

Smith, G.E. and Pear, T.H., *Shell-shock and Its Lessons*, Manchester, 1917.

Strahan, H., *The Outbreak of the First World War*, Oxford University Press, 2004.

Thompson, A., *Anzac Memories: Living with the Legend*, Oxford, 1994.

Tilton, M., *The Grey Battalion*, 2nd edn., Angus & Robertson, Sydney, 1934.

Times, *The Times Illustrated History of the War*, vol. VII. London, 1916.

Trahair, R.C. & J. G. Marshall, *Australian Psychoanalysis and Related Writings, 1884-1940, Annotated Bibliography*, La Trobe University Library, Melbourne, 1979.

Tyquin, M., *Gallipoli: The Medical War*, New South Wales University Press, Sydney, 1993.

——, *Little By Little: A Centenary History of the Royal Australian Army Medical Corps*, Australian Military History Publications, Sydney, 2003.

——, *Sir Neville Howse: Australia's First Victoria Cross Winner*, Oxford University Press, Melbourne, 1999.

Young, A., *The Harmony of Illusions: Inventing Post-Traumatic Stress Disorder*, Princeton, 1995.

Waite, F., *The New Zealanders at Gallipoli*, Whitcombe & Tombs, Auckland, 1921.

Walker, A. S., *Clinical Problems of the War*, Australia War Memorial, Canberra, 1952. Volume I in Series 5 (Medical) *Australia in the War of 1939-1945*.

Williams, J., *Anzacs, the Media and the Great War*, New South Wales University Press, Sydney, 1999.

Winter, D., *Death's Men: Soldiers of the Great War*, Penguin, Melbourne, 1979.

Index